WHAT ARE *YOUR* REASONS FOR QUITTING?

1. Smoking is bad for my health.
2. It makes my clothes, hair, home, and office smell bad.
3. I get out of breath more easily, and it hurts my athletic performance.
4. I spend too much money on cigarettes.
5. I feel that others disapprove of my smoking.
6. I worry that smoking may be a health risk to my friends and family.
7. I have more frequent colds, coughs, and sore throats.
8. I don't want to set a bad example for my children.
9. Smoking has hurt my friendships and hindered my romantic relationships.

WHATEVER YOUR REASONS, WHEN THE DRAWBACKS BEGIN TO ADD UP, TURN TO *THE NO-NAG, NO-GUILT, DO-IT-YOUR-OWN-WAY GUIDE TO QUITTING SMOKING*

THE NO-NAG, NO-GUILT, DO-IT-YOUR-OWN-WAY GUIDE TO QUITTING SMOKING

Tom Ferguson, M.D.

Chief Researcher: Gail M. Schmidt

BALLANTINE BOOKS • NEW YORK

A Ballantine Book
Published by The Random House Publishing Group
Copyright © 1987 by Tom Ferguson, M.D.
Introduction Copyright © 1988 by Tom Ferguson, M.D.

Published in the United States by Ballantine Books, an imprint of The Random House Publishing Group, a division of Random House, Inc., New York, and simultaneously in Canada by Random House of Canada Limited, Toronto. This book, or parts thereof, may not be reproduced in any form without permission.

The information this book contains is the result of a careful review of the medical literature. However, new information is constantly becoming available and individual reactions to specific treatments and methods vary widely from person to person. Thus the author and publisher strongly urge each reader to consult with his or her physician before acting on any of the information contained herein. The author and publisher specifically disclaim responsibility for any adverse effect or unforeseen consequences resulting from the implementation of any information mentioned in this book.

Library of Congress Catalog Card Number: 87-2578

ISBN 0-345-35578-4

This edition published by arrangement with G. P. Putnam's Sons, a division of the Putnam Publishing Group, Inc.

Manufactured in the United States of America

First Ballantine Books Edition: January 1989

OPM   29   28   27   26

To health-concerned smokers everywhere,
who *do* care about their health
and *do* want to take more control of their smoking—
in their own way and in their own time.

ACKNOWLEDGMENTS

I'm deeply grateful to the hundreds of health-concerned smokers and successful ex-smokers who volunteered so much of their time to tell us what should be included in *The No Nag, No Guilt, Do-It-Your-Own-Way Guide to Quitting Smoking*.

It was my Yale Medical School professor, Richard Selzer—physician, teacher, and writer *par excellence*—who planted the seed for this book ten years ago when he gently suggested that I take a close look at my own beliefs about smoking.

I owe a special debt of gratitude to Dr. Jerome Schwartz of Davis, California, one of our most respected smoking researchers, who invited me to join an American Cancer Society work group in discussing how the principles of self-care might be applied to smoking. The first rough outline for *The No Nag, No Guilt, Do-It-Your-Own-Way Guide to Quitting Smoking* came out of that meeting. Jerry, who recently completed a review of the scientific smoking literature of the past ten years for the National Cancer Institute, also gave us invaluable suggestions on an early draft of the manuscript.

Special thanks go to my friends Joe and Teresa Graedon, authors of *The People's Pharmacy* books and the syndicated column of the same name. The Graedons have pioneered a genuinely empowering kind of self-care writing. *The No Nag, No Guilt, Do-It-Your-Own-Way Guide to Quitting Smoking* has benefited from their comments, as has its author from their warm and supportive friendship.

I'm grateful for the cooperation of the always cheerful staff of the Department of Health and Human Services Office on Smoking and Health in Rockville, Maryland. They provided access to a researcher's dream of materials on smoking. With their help, researcher Gail Schmidt and I were able to review more than 5,000 scientific papers and abstracts on smoking and health.

I was fortunate indeed to receive the generous help of a number of the nation's top smoking researchers, smoking educators, and other medical experts in making sure that the factual information in this book was accurate and up-to-date. These include (in alphabetical order):

Russell Glasgow, Ph.D., Research Scientist, Oregon Research Institute, Eugene, Oregon.

Toni Goldfarb, Ph.D., Editor, *Medical Abstracts*, Teaneck, New Jersey.

Irving Goldstein, M.D., Professor of Urology, New England Male Reproductive Center, Boston University Medical School.

Ellen R. Gritz, Ph.D., Director, Division of Cancer Control, Jonsson Comprehensive Cancer Center, University of California, Los Angeles, California.

Neil E. Grunberg, Ph.D., Associate Professor of Medical Psychology, Uniformed Services University of Health Sciences, Bethesda, Maryland.

Sheldon Saul Hendler, M.D., Instructor, University of California School of Medicine, San Diego; Attending Internist, Mercy Hospital and Medical Center, San Diego, California.

Edward Lichtenstein, Professor of Psychology, University of Oregon, Eugene, Oregon; Research Scientist, Oregon Research Institute, Eugene, Oregon.

Karen Monaco and Shane McDermott, National Office of the American Lung Association, New York, New York.

Kenneth R. Pelletier, Ph.D., Associate Professor of Behavioral Medicine, University of California School of Medicine, San Francisco, California.

Olvide F. Pomerleau, Ph.D., Director, and Cynthia S. Pomerleau, Ph.D., Senior Research Associate, Behavioral Medicine Program, University of Michigan School of Medicine, Ann Arbor, Michigan.

Michael A. H. Russell, FRCP, FRCPSYCH, Addiction Research Unit, Institute of Psychiatry, London.

Victor J. Schoenbach, Ph.D., Assistant Professor, School of Public Health, University of North Carolina, Chapel Hill, North Carolina.

Saul Shiffman, Assistant Professor of Psychology, University of Pittsburgh, Pittsburgh, Pennsylvania.

S. Leonard Syme, Ph.D., Professor of Epidemiology, School of Public Health, University of California, Berkeley, California.

A number of other friends and colleagues provided important information, advice, and support:

Don Ardell provided a number of useful suggestions which were incorporated in the paperback edition.

Sheryl MacLaughlin decided to quit smoking in the midst of our interview and gave me a blow-by-blow account of her own quitting process. Michael Maguire, a successful quitter, described how everything may seem to go wrong in the weeks after you quit.

Charlotte Sheedy, a very special literary agent, got the project off to a good start and saw it through to a successful conclusion.

I am particularly grateful to the many people at G. P. Putnam's Sons who worked so hard to bring this book into the world:

Adrienne Ingrum—who took the ball and ran with it.

Anton Mueller—who made it a pleasure to work out the final details.

Mary Kurtz—who copyedited the manuscript with an eagle eye and a lively, perceptive intelligence.

Christine Schillig—who was my collaborator from the very beginning of this project. She served triple-duty—as an able and enthusiastic editor and advisor, as a health-concerned smoker in the research stage, and as a successful quitter as *The No Nag, No Guilt, Do-It-Your-Own-Way Guide to Quitting Smoking* neared completion. From the first time we discussed it, Chris's belief in the book never wavered.

Special thanks to the enthusiastically professional people at Ballantine Books who believed that a paperback edition would get this information into the hands of those who need it most:

Cheryl Woodruff, who first brought the book to Ballantine's attention.

Mary Ann Eckels, the editor who nursed the book—and its author—through the long production procedure.

Nora Reichard, a copy editor with a steady hand and a clear eye.

Asher Kingsley, who contributed a superb cover design.

Carol Fass and her staff, who worked long and hard to get the word out.

I'd like to express my profound gratitude to my chief researcher, Gail M. Schmidt, R.N., who put in countless hours and endless energy over the three years it took to research and write *The No Nag, No Guilt, Do-It-Your-Own-Way Guide to Quitting Smoking*. Without her help, this project would simply not have been possible.

Finally, I'd like to offer a very special thank-you to my wife, Meredith, and daughter, Adrienne, for their continuing love, support, and understanding during the many months this book was in process.

AUTHOR'S NOTE

Over the past ten years, an extraordinary number of people have contributed in one way or another to my ongoing efforts to provide the most useful available self-care information to the people who need it. Some provided inspiration and ideas, some their time and effort, others their love and encouragement. To all, my sincere appreciation and grateful thanks.

Wallace and Helen Ferguson
Fergus McLean
Kirpal Kaur Khalsa
George and Cynthia Mitchell
Michael Castleman
Carole Pisarczyk
The staff, writers, and subscribers of *Medical Self-Care* magazine

• • •

Lee Ammidon
Norma Ashby
J. Baldwin
Ginger Barber
Barlow Printing
Laurie Basch

Herbert Benson
Joan Borysenko
The Boston Women's Health Book Collective
Stewart Brand
Paul Bresnik
Bill and Peggy Brevoort
Mark Bricklin
John Brockman
Tom Bryan
Rick Carlson and Brooke Newman
Dede Clark
Norman Cousins
Betty and Ed Dreiss
Dean Edell
Les Edwards

Lewis and Brandy Engel
The Esalen Institute
Joni Evans
Marion Ferguson
Neshama Franklin
James Fries
Ann Godoff
Dan Goleman
Roger Gould
Dan Green
Doug and Karen Greene
Sadja Greenwood
Green Gulch Farm
Eileen Growald
Joel Guren
The Haight-Ashbury Free Clinic
T. George Harris
Ruth Hapgood
Bobbie Hasselbring
Bill Hettler
Mary Howell
Roger Hoffman
Ivan Illich
Charles Inlander
Ricky Jacobs
Howard Jacobson
Alberta Jacoby
Karen Johnson
Don Kemper
Kirpal Singh Khalsa
Ken Kreger
Michael Lerner
Lowell Levin
Stephen and Ondrea Levine
Amy Lipton and Ed Quinn
Steven Locke
Sheridan and Perry Lorenz
Pamela and Michael Maguire
Neal Miller
Grant Mitchell

Greg and Betsey Mitchell
Kent and Donna Mitchell
Kirk Mitchell
Mark Mitchell
Scott and Brenda Mitchell
Todd Mitchell
Michael Murphy
John Naisbitt
The National Wellness Conference at the University of Wisconsin, Stevens Point, Wisconsin
The National Women's Health Network
Marion Nestle
Wendy Nicholson
Nori and Jacquetta Nisbet
Cindy Ohama
Dean Ornish
Fran Pitlick
Lila Purinton
Dan Rather
Rachel Naomi Remen
Frank Riessman
Robert Rodale
Tim Rumsey
Eva Salber
Rachel Sanborn
Albert Schweitzer
Keith W. Sehnert
Jim Silberman
David S. Sobel
Summit Books
Angelica Thieriot
John Travis
Kerry Tremain
Don Vickery
The *Whole Earth Catalog*
The Yale University School of Medicine
Stewart and Beth Yudofsky

CONTENTS

ON DOING IT *YOUR* WAY

You're a smoker, and over the last few months and years, your habit has become a real burden.

Back when you started smoking, it seemed fun, sexy, and smart. Now it makes you feel guilty and ashamed.

You always knew your habit might cost you a few months or years of life. But it's now starting to cost you your friends. And you're afraid it may someday cost you your job.

You feel guiltier than ever about your smoking. Yet it's such a useful tool, such a good friend, that you are in despair at the thought of being forced to give it up.

Not that you *want* to be a smoker all your life. You *do* want to quit eventually. You're almost ready, but you're not quite sure.

Welcome, friend. We speak your language here. *The No-Nag, No-Guilt, Do-It-Your-Own-Way Guide to Quitting Smoking* was written with you in mind.

The No-Nag, No-Guilt, Do-It-Your-Own-Way Guide to Quitting Smoking book grew out of an invitation to advise the American Cancer Society how they might best encourage smokers to quit on their own. I suggested they start by asking smokers what kinds of information they— the smokers—would find most useful. I was astounded to find that no one had ever thought to ask.

We asked two hundred health-concerned smokers what kind of information *they'd* find most useful in taking control of their habit in the way they saw fit.* *The No-Nag, No-Guilt, Do-It-Your-Own-Way Guide to Quitting Smoking* presents the information those smokers asked for. It's presented it in the way *they* wanted it presented—a respectful, nonblaming way that leaves the final decision up to each individual smoker. The smokers in our survey said that most quit-smoking books just made them feel guilty. *The No-Nag, No-Guilt, Do-It-Your-Own-Way Guide to Quitting Smoking* is designed to *expand* your range of options and to *support* your sense of yourself as a responsible, competent, powerful person.

Although our main goal has been to produce a book smokers could use on their own, *The No-Nag, No-Guilt, Do-It-Your-Own-Way Guide to Quitting Smoking* has also been adopted as a text by smoking education programs across the country. Many nonsmokers have given this book to friends and family members. Employers provide copies for their employees. Smokers say it's the first book on the subject that told them something they didn't already know. Others have thanked us for writing a hopeful, positive book that didn't make them feel guilty.

The take-home lesson of *The No-Nag, No-Guilt, Do-It-Your-Own-Way Guide to Quitting Smoking* is this: **There's only one way to quit smoking: You have to do it yourself.** While there *are* some extremely powerful tools and techniques to help you accomplish your goal— you'll find them listed in the chapters that follow—none of them will "make" you a nonsmoker. It's much like

*For details of our smoker survey, see p. 283.

building a house: no saw or hammer can do it for you, but you can learn to master the tools required to do the job.

We suggest you start by reading the chapters that follow. Please *do* underline, take notes, or turn down pages to mark the tools and techniques that have a special appeal. After you've finished the book, we suggest you review the sections you've marked and begin planning your own self-designed quitting program. We suggest that you combine at least half a dozen, and ideally a dozen or more of these tools and techniques. Studies show that the *more* strategies you combine, the more likely you are to become a permanent nonsmoker.

Once you've chosen the techniques you'd like to use, get out your calendar and begin setting some specific goals. You don't need to set a quitting date right away. Wait till it feels right. You might choose to spend two or three months getting an exercise program up and running. You might want to begin by recruiting a key support person. You might decide to begin by upgrading your stress control skills. Or you may decide to use our guidelines for controlled smoking to cut your number of cigarettes per day in half within the next month.

In addition to setting such short-term goals, you may want to start thinking about possible quitting dates. Give yourself permission to choose a quitting date several weeks or months in the future. Give yourself as much time as you need. Don't let anyone push you into attempting to quit before you feel ready.

You're going to do it *your* way. And don't let anyone tell you different.

Good health and good luck,

Tom Ferguson, M.D.
Austin, Texas

Basic Information

1

The Smoker's Dilemma: What We Learned from 200 Smokers

In the course of writing *The No-Nag, No-Guilt, Do-It-Your-Own-Way Guide to Quitting Smoking*, researcher Gail Schmidt and I interviewed over 200 health-concerned smokers. One hundred of these smokers completed a detailed questionnaire. (For the results of that survey, see *Appendix V.*)

We thought we might find these smokers blasé. Instead, we found a great deal of confusion and torment. "Sometimes I just sit there in front of my mirror with a cigarette in my mouth and watch myself inhaling that poison gas," one smoker lamented. "I know that if I was in a concentration camp and someone tried to make me do that, I'd want to *kill* them."

These smokers told us that they felt confused and conflicted about the role smoking plays in their lives. On the one hand, they see smoking as a pleasant, relaxing, and helpful personal ritual that provides them with undeniable benefits. On the other hand, they know it increases their risk of ill health and will, in all likelihood, shorten their lives. As one woman smoker put it, "It's like being

in love with a man who's no good. You *know* you're a
fool. But you just can't help it.''

The Rise of the
Health-concerned Smoker

We had expected denial of the negative effects of smoking. Instead, we found that most of the smokers we interviewed *over*estimated the negative effects of cigarettes
on their health.[1] When we asked health-concerned smokers to estimate the number of years of life they would
gain if they quit, the average estimate was 14.6 years.
This is roughly twice what experts project. Some smokers thought that smoking would cost them as much as 35
years of life. "If I could quit today, I'd live to see my
daughter's grandchildren," one woman told us. "If I
don't, I'll be lucky to see my own."

Why Smokers Feel Guilty

Far from denying the negative health effects of their habit,
the smokers we interviewed felt intensely guilty about it.
Forty-nine percent said they felt more guilty about their
smoking now than they did a few years ago. And when
asked to rate exactly *how* guilty they felt, smokers rated
themselves at 7.0 on a scale of 10 (with 10 being extremely guilty and 1 being not at all guilty).

Those who had tried and failed to quit felt particularly
guilty: "After I go to bed at night and I'm drifting
through that dreamy place just before sleep, I always
think, 'I'm *not* going to smoke tomorrow. I'm *not* going
to do this to myself any more,' " one smoker told us. "I
think of how bad it is for me, how bad it is for my two
sons. And I feel this big burst of resolve. But then, first

thing in the morning, I grind the coffee, I pour myself a fresh cup, I take that first sip, and I reach for a cigarette.''

Those who have children at home feel guiltiest of all: ''Ever since my daughter started to talk, she's told me she wished I didn't smoke,'' one young father told us. '' 'Your smoke stinks, Daddy,' she'll say. 'It makes me want to throw up. I can't breathe when you're blowing all that smoke around.' And even though I *know* it's hurting her, I'll sit there in the house and smoke anyway. I *really* hate myself for that.''

Secret Smokers

Some smokers feel so guilty they go underground with their habit. We interviewed a number of smokers who hide their smoking from their spouse, their boss, their children, or other friends and family members. Like secret drinkers, they go to great lengths to shroud their habit in a cloak of deception. Some people smoke at work while denying at home that they smoke at all. Others smoke only in secret.

Most Smokers *Do* Respect Nonsmokers' Rights

We expected resentment toward nonsmokers. And we did find some. But we also found that within the last few years, smokers have become *much* more sensitive to the effects of their smoking on their nonsmoking friends. Seventy-five percent of the smokers we interviewed said that they were now more likely to refrain from smoking while in the presence of nonsmokers. Ninety-one percent said they are now more likely to ask permission to smoke while visiting a nonsmoking friend.

A recent Gallup Poll found that 85 percent of nonsmokers *and 62 percent of smokers* agreed that smokers should refrain from smoking in the presence of nonsmokers. The same survey found that 80 percent of current smokers, 89 percent of former smokers, and 92 percent of nonsmokers felt that smoking should be either regulated or banned at the workplace.[2]

Smoking as a Blue-Collar Custom

Among many groups, especially the younger, more affluent, and the better educated, smoking has become a distinct social stigma. A 1985 study published by the Centers for Disease Control found that while 40 percent of white women who had been high-school dropouts smoked, among their classmates who graduated from college, only 15 percent were smokers. About 50 percent of men with blue-collar jobs smoke, compared to 26 percent among

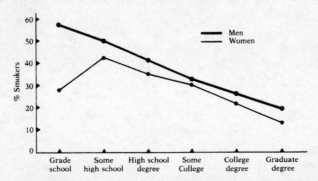

Figure 1-1 Smoking Prevalence by Education
Dotted bars indicate men; slashed bars, women. Data is for white Americans; compiled 1981–1983.[5]

professional men. Between 1978 and 1980, all social groups but one—blue-collar women—decreased their smoking rate.[3]

A 1984 Harris Poll found that although 32 percent of those who had not graduated from high school were smokers, the figure for college graduates was only 19 percent. The same poll found that among adults with household incomes under $7,500, 34 percent smoked. For adults with household incomes over $50,000, the figure was 18 percent.[4]

"There's not a single person among our close friends who smokes any more," a nonsmoking San Francisco psychologist told us. "Not a single one. Yet when I attend local meetings of a fishermen's group I belong to, there are a great many smokers, most of them older men who work at blue-collar jobs." In effect, one might say that the connotations associated with smoking a generation ago—those of style, urbanity, social standing—have been reversed in our own time.

Smokers as a Persecuted Minority

This widespread change in attitude toward smoking makes many smokers feel like a persecuted minority. Fully 40 percent of our subjects told us that their smoking had been a problem in their romantic relationships. For 12 percent, it had been a serious one. For some, it had been the principal factor in the breakup of the relationship. "There's no question about it," one woman told us. "Chris and I would be together today if I'd been able to quit. He was just dead set against marrying a smoker."

Antismoker Discrimination in the Workplace

Many of the smokers we interviewed expressed concern that their habit might interfere with career success. "The shift supervisor at my hospital doesn't like nurses who smoke," one nurse told us. Her supervisor is not alone. One recent survey of 529 managers found that smoking was cited as the number one "annoying personal habit" among employees. Smoking was cited more than twice as frequently than any other behavior.[6]

Dr. William Weis of the Albers Business School at Seattle University has estimated that it costs the average employer up to $4,500 per year to hire a smoker. Weis bases this on the following estimates:

- increased absenteeism (smokers are absent 45 to 57 percent more often);

- increased risk of death (smokers are 70 to 270 percent more likely to die);

- increased accident rates (smokers are roughly twice as likely to have accidents);

- decreased productivity (smokers waste an estimated 35 minutes more of each business day than nonsmokers);

- increased property damage and maintenance (smokers increase maintenance expenses by an estimated $500 per year);

- decreased morale among nonsmokers (nonsmokers who work around smokers exhibit respiratory changes equivalent to those found in persons who smoke one to ten cigarettes per day).

Weis suggests that cost-conscious employers stop hiring smokers and prohibit smoking on company property. Many employers have done exactly that.[7]

Smokers Want More Control

The great majority of the smokers we interviewed said they'd like to increase their control over their habit. Ninety percent of those who smoked more than ten cigarettes per day told us they'd like to have more control over their smoking. Ninety-four percent of current smokers say they'd like to quit. Eighty-four percent have made serious attempts to do so. Sixty percent have quit at some time in the past, but started smoking again. Of those who have quit, seventy-six percent stayed off cigarettes for a week or more, while twenty-eight percent stayed off for more than a year.

Smokers as Outcasts

One of our subjects—we'll call her Susan Saunders—was particularly eloquent about the smoker's dilemma. At thirty-eight, Susan owns her own design agency. "Having a cigarette after a meal has always been the most relaxing time of my day," she recalls. For nearly as long as she can remember, Susan has used cigarettes to relax, to take work breaks, and to help her concentrate on important jobs.

"There was a time not long ago when cigarettes were considered a necessary part of the good life," she says, carefully touching her ash to the center of the crystal ashtray on the coffee table in her beachfront condominium. "Smoking used to have class. Humphrey Bogart used to reach for a Chesterfield with the kind of assurance you see today only when somebody reaches for a

Perrier. Today being a smoker is the kiss of death: It keeps you from getting kissed. And if you're single, like I am, that's death.''

Susan has seen nonsmokers' attitudes toward smoking change dramatically. "Friends who used to bring me an ashtray now have cute little No Smoking signs on their front door. It used to be that a person's smoking habits were her own business. Now it's become a big public issue. And the worst thing of all is the new evidence that cigarette smoke is harmful to *non*smokers.'' She shakes her head sadly and blows smoke up at the ceiling. "It's one thing to cause a friend a little mild discomfort. It's quite another to produce growth retardation in a friend's unborn baby.''

Nonsmokers Have Become More Assertive

In addition to their own feelings of confusion and guilt, smokers must deal with an increasing number of anti-smoking messages and a much more open display of anti-smoking sentiment. Sixty-eight percent of our subjects said that nonsmokers in restaurants are now more likely to complain about their smoking.

Such pressure can be disconcerting for smokers. San Francisco author Paul Erdman was recently dining at a very expensive restaurant. He paid the $300 check and lit up a cigar. "They threw us out,'' he recalls. "The chef came out, the owner arrived—everyone—and they threw us out. They would have pitched us through the window if they could have. I guess that qualifies as social pressure.''[8]

Some smokers fear that antismoking sentiment may grow even more intense: Antismoking advocates in some cities have used spray cans to "zap'' smokers.[9]

A Los Angeles man was stabbed when he refused to put out his cigarette. Another smoker was shot by a New York transit policeman in a dispute over smoking.[10] A respected Seattle physician was recently arrested for altering billboards that carried cigarette ads. To the slogan "Camel Lights: It's a Whole New World," he had added "of cancer." He also changed the slogan "Winston: America's Best" to "Winston: America's Death."[11]

Nonsmokers have become much more assertive collectively as well. Within recent years thirty-nine states—as well as hundreds of local communities—have passed laws prohibiting or limiting smoking in public places.[12] The National Association of Insurance Commissioners recently adopted a resolution urging insurance companies to raise smokers' insurance premiums by roughly 50 percent.[13]

"It's all getting to be a real burden for those of us who still smoke," Susan Saunders says. "Today's 'scarlet letter' is the big red S we smokers feel we wear around our necks. I recently saw a lapel button that says it all: 'Smoking is always having to say you're sorry.' "

Why Smokers Can't Quit

Why don't these tortured smokers quit? The necessary period of withdrawal poses a powerful barrier. Eighty-four percent of the smokers we interviewed told us that if they could find a method that would make it possible for them to quit without experiencing the unpleasantness of withdrawal, they would be much more likely to quit.

But while withdrawal is a major reason why smokers don't quit, it is not the only one. *The smokers we sur-*

veyed told us that in addition to preventing withdrawal symptoms, smoking provides them with some very positive benefits. When we asked smokers to list the perceived benefits smoking provides, they ranked them in the following order:

1. Smoking helps me deal with stressful situations.
2. Smoking provides a pleasant and enjoyable break from work.
3. Smoking helps me unwind and relax.
4. (tie) Smoking helps me deal with painful or unpleasant situations;
4. (tie) Smoking prevents unpleasant withdrawal symptoms.
5. Smoking helps me deal with an overstimulating environment.
6. I enjoy the physical sensation of lighting and handling a cigarette.
7. Smoking keeps me from feeling bored.
8. Smoking increases my enjoyment of pleasant experiences.
9. Smoking helps me feel comfortable in social situations.
10. Helps me to concentrate.

Planning to Quit

Eighty-six percent of the smokers we interviewed said they believed that they *would* quit. But they emphasized that one must choose one's own time to quit, and must do so at a time when life is less stressful and support for quitting is available.

How to Help a Health-Concerned Smoker

Smokers gave very low marks to their friends and family members' efforts to help them take control of their smoking. They felt that the principal strategy used by most antismokers was to nag the smokers closest to them into quitting. But this tactic frequently has just the opposite effect. A dozen smokers responded with virtually the same words: "Unsympathetic nagging just makes me smoke *more*." Smokers suggest that concerned friends adopt the following strategies:

- Don't nag, insult, or try to shame the smoker into quitting.
- Let your smoking friends know that you value them as people, even though you may disapprove of their smoking.
- Learn to listen nonjudgmentally. Try to understand what benefits the smoker derives from this very seductive habit. Try to see the problem through the smoker's eyes.
- Praise the smoker for even the smallest efforts to cut down or quit.

(For a more detailed discussion of this topic, see *Appendix I: How to Help a Health-Concerned Smoker*.)

"Nonsmokers just don't understand," Saunders says, stubbing her Carlton out and lighting a new one. "I don't *need* to be told smoking is bad for me. I *know* that. I don't *need* to be told I ought to quit. What I need are some concrete, workable suggestions as to what my options are. What I need is support for the belief that I can do it. What I need most of all is lots and lots of help when I *do* decide to make the final break."

Full Disclosure

When we asked health-concerned smokers to rank the kinds of information they would find most useful in their efforts to take control of their smoking, they listed the following topics as most important:

1. How to *stay* a nonsmoker after you quit.
2. The most effective ways of quitting.
3. The most effective ways of cutting down.
4. Getting ready to quit: What smokers need to know.
5. Do smokers have special needs for vitamins?
6. What smoking does to a smoker's body.
7. How to tell whether you're a high- or low-risk smoker.
8. Dealing with weight gain after you quit.
9. What withdrawal symptoms smokers may encounter after they quit.
10. How to cut your smoking risk through better stress management.

In the chapters that follow, we have done our best to provide health-concerned smokers with the information they said they wanted.

The Only Equation in this Book

I dislike giving mathematical formulas in a book of this nature, but in this case, there is one very simple equation I would like to share with you.[14] This is an extremely useful equation because it gives health-concerned smokers an overview of the different steps they can take to reduce their smoking risk.

For current smokers, the risk of smoking-related illness or death may be represented as follows:

$$\text{Smoking-related Risk} = \frac{\text{Total Lifetime Dose} \times \text{Individual Risk Level}}{\text{Wellness Level}}$$

This equation suggests that you can cut your smoking-related risk by three different strategies:

- Cut or eliminate your dose of tobacco smoke (covered in chapters 6 through 12).
- Increase your wellness level (covered in chapter 5).
- Identify and cut your individual risk factors (covered in chapter 4).

You could, of course, reduce your smoking-related risks even more quickly by adopting two or three strategies at once.

• • •

Whether you smoke or not is *your choice*. But to make that choice effectively you must consider your alternatives, and the benefits and hazards of each.

We can't promise easy answers or magical solutions. In smoking, as in most areas of life, there are no miracle cures or quick fixes. There are, however, some pretty powerful tools, many of them not widely known.

We've done our best to present the facts about smoking from an impartial, no-fault point of view. Our three years of research on the subject have convinced us that as a health-concerned smoker, you *can* take more control of your smoking. Your spouse, your family, your friends, your physician, and others in your home community *can* provide important tools, caring, and support. *But the key to success is for you to take primary responsibility to make the changes you desire.*

In the chapters that follow, we'll provide guidelines for putting together your own tailor-made smoking control program. Planning and implementing that program is up to you.

2

Smoking as a Psychological Tool

Let's imagine for a moment that scientists had discovered a new psychoactive drug—let's call it "Drug X"—that could:

- help you deal with stress;
- help you calm down when you were feeling tense;
- help pep you up when you were feeling lethargic;
- help you concentrate more effectively;
- make it easier to control unpleasant feelings;
- produce a mild state of euphoria.

Suppose too that this new drug could help you fine-tune your nervous system to achieve exactly the mood you desired—larger doses would help you relax, while smaller doses would pep you up and help you focus on the task at hand. And on top of all that, suppose that "Drug X" could help you shed excess pounds—without dieting.

"Drug X" may sound like a drug company's dream, but there *is* such a drug. In the United States alone users take well over *10 billion doses per day*. The drug, of course, is nicotine.

Why Smokers Smoke

Nicotine is the only known psychoactive ingredient in tobacco smoke. Addicted smokers smoke for one principal reason—to get their accustomed doses of nicotine. As the respected British smoking researcher M.A.H. Russell has written, "If it were not for the nicotine in tobacco smoke, people would be little more inclined to smoke cigarettes than they are to blow bubbles or light sparklers."[1] Indeed, smokers have found nicotine-free cigarettes so unacceptable that researchers have sometimes been unable to use them for research purposes.[2]

More Than an Addiction

Most smokers realize that smoking is addictive—that is to say, when a habitual smoker stops smoking, he or she is likely to experience such unpleasant symptoms as irritability, sensitivity to sounds, light, and touch, and sudden, irrational mood changes. Many nonsmokers think that smokers smoke only to avoid such withdrawal symptoms. But recent research shows that in addition to preventing withdrawal, nicotine seems to provide a surprising variety of desirable psychological effects.

British smoking researchers Ashton and Stepney first suggested in 1982 that nicotine serves the smoker as a very powerful psychological tool.[3] It is these psychological benefits combined with the unpleasant symptoms that may result from cessation that make it so difficult for smokers to quit.

The smokers we interviewed told us that avoiding

withdrawal symptoms was only a *small part* of the reason they smoke. They smoke primarily for the *positive effects* smoking provides. Until recently, little attention has been paid to these positive effects, but we are increasingly gaining important insights into the psychopharmacology of nicotine. And an understanding of the mechanisms by which nicotine provides positive psychological effects can be a valuable tool for smokers who wish to control their smoking behavior.

200 Nicotine "Hits" Per Day

The average smoker takes ten puffs per cigarette. For the pack-a-day smoker, this works out to about 200 puffs per day. Each "hit" of nicotine reaches the smoker's brain within seven seconds, about twice as fast as a syringeful of heroin injected into a vein. (Heroin must pass through a good part of the body's systemic circulatory system before reaching the brain, while the nicotine-rich blood from the lungs passes directly to the brain.)

Once nicotine enters the brain, it appears to mimic the action of the neurotransmitter acetylcholine and to stimulate production of a number of the brain's most powerful chemical messengers: epinephrine (adrenaline), norepinephrine, dopamine, arginine, vasopressin, and beta-endorphine. Acetylcholine is involved in alertness, pain reduction, learning, and memory. Norepinephrine regulates alertness and arousal. Dopamine is part of the brain's pleasure mechanism. Beta-endorphine, which has been called the brain's own natural analgesic, can reduce anxiety and pain.[4] The net effect is a temporary improvement in brain chemistry that is experienced by the smoker as enhanced pleasure, decreased anxiety, and a state of alert relaxation.

As a result of this positive reinforcement many dozens

of times per day, smoking becomes thoroughly interwoven into every nook and cranny of a smoker's life. These recent discoveries about the positive effects of smoking help explain why the smoking habit holds its victims in such a tenacious grip.[5]

The smokers we interviewed told us that smoking helped them concentrate, kept them from being bored, and helped reduce the perceived level of tension in their lives. In addition, smoking helped them cope with an overstimulating environment, gave them positive pleasure, helped them relax, reduced their feelings of distress, helplessness, and loneliness, helped them keep their weight down, and made them feel more at ease in social situations. Understandably, these substantial benefits would be difficult to give up. But there are even more.

They told us that smoking also helped to provide a quick burst of energy when they were feeling tired, provided them with enjoyable tactile sensations, and helped them work and concentrate more effectively. And these effects were not only observed by the smokers we interviewed; they have been studied and described by many researchers. It is now a well-documented fact that *smoking helps smokers control their moods*.

How Smoking Serves as a "Mood Thermostat"

The secret to smoking's ability to control moods is its capacity to regulate the level of arousal of key parts of the brain and central nervous system.

First, nicotine helps set a smoker's general level of arousal (GLA), which is determined by a part of the brain called the reticular formation. The neurotransmitters through which most nerve impulses are transmitted within

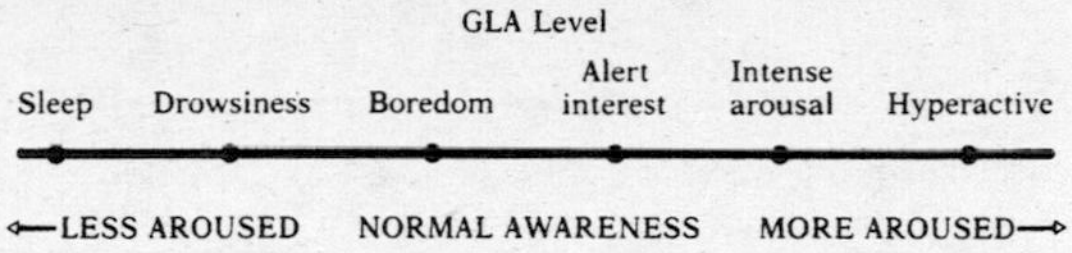

GLA Level

| Sleep | Drowsiness | Boredom | Alert interest | Intense arousal | Hyperactive |

←—LESS AROUSED   NORMAL AWARENESS   MORE AROUSED—→

Figure 2-1 The General Level of Arousal (GLA) Scale

the reticular formation are mediated by the neurotransmitter acetylcholine (ACh). Nicotine modifies nerve transmission involving ACh and other neurotransmitters at the junctions between nerve cells. Thus nicotine can "tune" a smoker's GLA either up or down, producing either stimulation or relaxation.

The smokers we interviewed reported that they use nicotine not only as a stimulant but as a relaxant as well. Smoking is thus used to increase arousal in periods of boredom and to decrease it in periods of excessive stress. When smokers wish to achieve a stimulating effect, they take short, quick puffs. This produces a *low* level of blood nicotine, which stimulates nerve transmission. When they wish to relax, they take deep drags, which produce *high* levels. This depresses the passage of nerve impulses, producing a mild sedative effect. Ashton and Stepney suggest that there is an "optimal" nicotine dose for any given activity, and that smokers unconsciously regulate their smoking patterns in order to obtain this optimal dose: "It appears that each smoker can, by varying his smoking style, figuratively slide up and down his nicotine dose-response curve to obtain the stimulant or depressant effect he requires in the prevailing circumstances."[6]

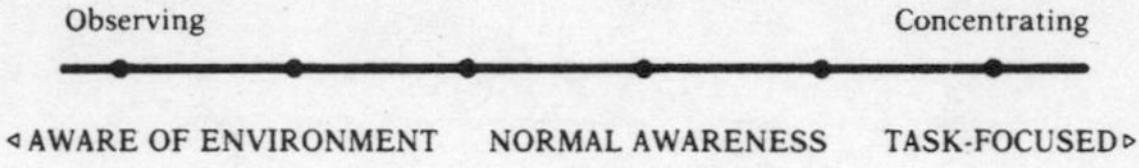

Observing   Concentrating

◄ AWARE OF ENVIRONMENT   NORMAL AWARENESS   TASK-FOCUSED ►

Figure 2-2 The "Attention Thermostat"

How Smoking Improves Attention and Performance

Nicotine also serves as an "attention thermostat"—it helps determine our response to environmental stimuli. It promotes "selective attention" and thus aids in certain kinds of learning and improves certain kinds of memory. Nicotine seems to help smokers feel less overwhelmed by disruptive or distracting stimulation in their environment and makes it easier for them to concentrate on the task at hand.

The "attention thermostat" effect is mediated through the limbic system of the brain. The principal transmitters in the limbic system are adrenaline and dopamine. Both are influenced by nicotine.

When the thermostat is turned to the "nonselective response" end of the attention thermostat, a person becomes jumpy. Every little environmental stimulus is much more likely to be experienced as distracting. When it is tuned to the "selective response" end, the person is capable of focusing on the task at hand and ignoring a wide variety of distracting environmental stimuli.

For any task, there is probably an optimal point on the attention thermostat. By selecting the desired nicotine dose, smokers can choose the state of mind most suited to an activity. Smoking thus provides smokers with the ability to improve concentration and increase their powers of vigilance and attention.

Smoking Helps Maintain Alertness for Boring Tasks

Some of the most striking benefits of smoking are observed when a smoker is faced with a boring, repetitive task. In a British study subjects were asked to watch for pauses in the movement of the hand of a clock. Subjects were paid for each pause they noticed. The performance of the smokers allowed to smoke continued at a high level throughout the sixty-minute test period. The performance of both deprived smokers *and nonsmokers* deteriorated with time. Similar studies have yielded similar results.[7]

Smoking Improves Certain Types of Learning

There is substantial evidence that smoking affects learning and memory. Smoking apparently helps consolidate learned material into long-term memory, although smokers remember *less* "incidental" material—apparently because of their increased powers of concentration. Smoking helps them narrow their attention to the most important aspects of the task at hand.[8]

In one experiment, subjects were asked to name the ink color in which a number of color names were written. This is a potentially confusing task, since the ink color chosen was always different from the color named: The word "red" might be written in yellow ink, the word "blue" might be written in green ink, and so on. Nicotine helped smokers sort out the information more quickly. Even more surprising, *nicotine injections also resulted in improved performance in nonsmokers.*[9]

Smoking Helps Smokers Control Anger and Anxiety

Smoking can also help smokers control angry or anxious feelings. One study speculated that smoking may be used to attenuate these emotional responses through the depressant effects of nicotine on limbic arousal and punishment.[10]

Smoking can help the smoker deal with frustrations without actually becoming angry. As one smoker we interviewed put it, "When I get to the point where my job is driving me crazy and I just want to explode, I light up a cigarette. Cigarettes are my 'cork'—they help me keep the anger in."

This "corking" effect was beautifully demonstrated in one insightful study in which three groups (smokers allowed to smoke, nonsmokers, and deprived smokers) played a mechanical game on a machine that had been programmed to "cheat." The players found themselves in a situation much like that of "the hapless victim of the machine age whose coin fails to win him a drink in an automatic dispensing machine."

At the researcher's urging, all three groups continued to play. The smokers allowed to smoke simply shrugged off this unpleasant event. Their scores did not deteriorate. The net effect of smoking was to moderate their emotional reactions and to enhance their ability to concentrate on a task.[11] But both the nonsmokers and the deprived smokers became so angry that their scores fell. The researchers concluded that smoking provided smoking subjects with an increased ability to deal with conditions that might ordinarily disrupt their concentration.[12]

Smoking Helps Smokers Cope with Stress

Nicotine can help both humans and animals deal more effectively with stress. In test animals, nicotine injections reduce the disruption of behavior produced by such unpleasant stimuli as a shock or—for rats—the presence of a cat.[13] Nicotine injections also improve test animals' ability to perform a learned behavior under stressful conditions.[14] In addition, both aggressive feelings and jaw-clenching behavior in humans have been shown to be reduced by nicotine.[15]

Smoking Helps Smokers Deal with Pain

In a 1984 study, the effects of nicotine on the pain awareness of smokers were measured. The subjects were asked to immerse one hand in a container of ice water. They were asked to indicate the time when they first became aware of the pain (pain awareness threshold) and the time when they could no longer endure the pain (pain tolerance threshold). During some of the trials, the smokers smoked their usual brand of cigarettes. During other trials, they smoked zero-nicotine cigarettes. The researchers found that smoking the nicotine-containing cigarette dulled the smokers' awareness of pain. This and other studies suggest that nicotine can produce significant pain relief.[16].

Smoking Gives Smokers a Sense of Control

Strange as it may seem to nonsmokers, many of the smokers we spoke with said that cigarettes gave them a strong sense of control. This effect results from the extraordinary efficiency and speed with which smoking delivers a dose of the active substance to the brain. As stated earlier, each ''hit'' reaches the brain within seven seconds, providing instant gratification. The average smoker self-administers approximately 200 to 300 nicotine ''hits'' per day.

The smoker is in total control of the timing and the dose. Thus smoking gives smokers a great deal of control over their own nervous systems. As Christen and Cooper write, ''The person who has never smoked cannot possibly understand the depth of affective satisfaction derived from this habit.''[17]

●   ●   ●

In reviewing the existing studies, one can only conclude that in addition to its many well-known *harmful physical effects*—which will be described in detail in chapter 3—smoking provides smokers with an impressive range of *desirable psychological effects*. Smokers are obtaining these short-term psychological benefits at the cost of long-term physical hazards. This is an important key to the smoker's dilemma.

Smokers do *not* smoke just to avoid withdrawal. They smoke because of the very real benefits that smoking provides. Thus one strategy available to health-concerned smokers who wish to reduce their smoking risks would be to find other ways to achieve the same or similar benefits. (This approach will be covered in more detail in chapter 5.) It is also clear that virtually all psychological benefits, as well as virtually all of the unpleasant withdrawal symptoms, can be attributed to the presence or absence of nicotine. But nicotine itself, in the doses to which smokers are exposed, is, at the very least, considerably less harmful than the tars and carbon monoxide found in tobacco smoke.[18] Thus the health-concerned smoker may wish to explore the possibility of temporarily obtaining nicotine from nicotine gum or other nontobacco sources. (This approach is covered in greater detail in chapter 9.)

3

What Smoking Does to Your Body

Smoking is a major health hazard. There is now an exhaustive body of evidence—including hundreds of epidemiological, experimental, pathological, and clinical studies—to demonstrate that smoking increases the smoker's risk of death and illness from a wide variety of diseases.[1] The U.S. Surgeon General has called cigarette smoking "the chief preventable cause of death in our society."[2] The National Institute on Drug Abuse has estimated that in the U.S. alone, smoking is responsible for approximately 350,000 excess deaths per year.[3] Other estimates range as high as 540,000 deaths per year.[4]

Most smokers accept the fact that smoking is harmful, but many think of this risk as something like a game of roulette: They believe that each cigarette they smoke is like placing a bet. The "prize" is a heart attack, lung cancer, or some other disease. If your "number" comes up, you've had it, but if you are "lucky" and your number never comes up, you may avoid the hazardous effects of smoking altogether and live to a ripe old age totally unaffected by your smoking habit.

This is a serious misconception. *Every cigarette you smoke harms your body.* Here's a better analogy:

Suppose you lived near a chemical plant that emitted a number of toxic wastes that had seeped into the town's drinking water, so that every time you took a drink of water, it did a small amount of damage to your body. After you'd lived there for a few years, you might notice that you didn't have quite as much energy as you used to. And after five or ten years, you might notice that quite a few of the townspeople seemed to be getting ill with one thing or another.

In the same way, *every cigarette you smoke damages your body.* The more you smoke, the greater the damage. True, there have been people who lived into their seventies and eighties even though they smoked all their lives, but unless they were either extremely light smokers or did not inhale, they almost certainly suffered substantial physical impairment as the result of their smoking while they were alive. If they had not smoked, they would in all likelihood have lived even longer.

Smoking Risks—Rules of Thumb

- Lung cancer risk—increases roughly 50 to 100 percent for each cigarette you smoke per day.
- Heart disease risks—increases roughly 100 percent for each pack of cigarettes you smoke per day.
- Switching to filter-tip cigarettes reduces the risk of lung cancer roughly 20 percent, but does not affect the risk of heart disease.
- Smokers spend 27 percent more time in the hospital and more than twice as much time in intensive care units as nonsmokers.
- Each cigarette costs the smoker five to twenty minutes of life.
- A smoker is at twice the risk of dying before age sixty-five as a nonsmoker.[36]

Inside a Smoker's Body

Let's take a look at what happens inside your body each time you light up. You may be surprised to learn how quickly tobacco smoke can produce harmful effects.

EYES, NOSE, THROAT

- Within a few seconds of your first puff, irritating gases (formaldehyde, ammonia, hydrogen sulfide, and others) begin to work on sensitive membranes of your eyes, nose, and throat. They make your eyes water and your nose run. They irritate your throat. If you continue smoking, these irritating gases will eventually produce a smoker's cough. One of the reasons many smokers prefer menthol cigarettes is that menthol is an anesthetic that masks the smoker's perception of this irritation.[5]

- Continued smoking produces abnormal thickening in the membranes lining your throat. This thickening is accompanied by cellular changes that have been linked to throat cancer.[6]

**Why Smokers Frequently Experience
a Morning Cough**

Because you haven't smoked all night, the cilia in your bronchi, which were knocked out of action by the toxic effects of cigarette smoke the day before, begin to come to life and attempt to clear the accumulated mucus out of your air passages. This cleansing action brings up a thick yellow or yellow-green mucus, which triggers the cough reflex in the back of your throat.

LUNGS

- From your very first puff, the smoke begins to chip away at your lung's natural defenses. Continued exposure can completely paralyze the lungs' natural cleansing process.

- Your respiratory rate increases, forcing your lungs to work harder.

- Irritating gases produce chemical injury to the tissues of your lungs and the airways leading to the lungs. This speeds up the production of mucus and leads to an increased tendency to cough up sputum.

- This excess mucus serves as a breeding ground for a wide variety of bacteria and viruses. This makes you more susceptible to colds, flu, bronchitis, and other respiratory infections. And if you do come down with an infection, your body will be less able to fight it, because smoking impairs the ability of the white blood cells to resist invading organisms.

- The lining of your bronchi begins to thicken, predisposing you to cancers of the bronchi. Most lung cancers arise in the bronchial lining.

- Farther down, inside your lungs, the smoke weakens the free-roving scavenger cells that remove foreign particles from the air sacs of the lungs. Continued smoke exposure adversely affects elastin (the enzyme that keeps your lungs flexible), predisposing you to emphysema.

- Many of the compounds you inhale are deposited as a layer of sticky tar on the lining of your throat and bronchi and in the delicate air sacs of your lungs. A pack-a-day smoker pours about eight ounces—one full cup—of tar into his or her lungs each year. This tar is

rich in cancer-producing chemicals, including radioactive polonium 210.[7]

> EXPERIMENT: Breathe in a full mouthful of smoke,
> but don't inhale. Blow the smoke out through a
> clean white handkerchief. The amount of tar left on
> the handkerchief is roughly equivalent to the
> amount each puff leaves in your lungs.

HEART

- From the moment smoke reaches your lungs, your heart
  is forced to work harder. Your pulse quickens, forcing
  your heart to beat an extra 10 to 25 times per minute,
  as many as 36,000 additional times per day.

- Because of the irritating effect of nicotine and other
  components of tobacco smoke, your heartbeat is more
  likely to be irregular. This can contribute to cardiac
  arrhythmias, and many other serious coronary conditions, such as heart attack. A recent Surgeon General's
  report estimated that about 170,000 heart attacks each
  year are caused by smoking.

BLOOD VESSELS

- Your blood pressure increases by 10 to 15 percent, putting additional stress on your heart and blood vessels,
  increasing your risk of heart attack and stroke.

- Smoking increases your risk of vascular disease of the
  extremities. Severe cases may require amputation. This
  condition can produce pain and can increase your risk
  of blood clots in the lungs.

SKIN

- Smoking constricts the blood vessels in your skin, decreasing the delivery of life-giving oxygen to this vital organ. As the result of this decrease in blood flow, a smoker's skin becomes more susceptible to wrinkling. This decreased blood flow can be a special problem in people who suffer from chronically cold hands and/or feet (Raynaud's Syndrome).

- Smokers are at particularly high risk for a medical syndrome called "smoker's face," which is characterized by deep lines around the corners of the mouth and eyes, a gauntness of facial features, a grayish appearance of the skin, and certain abnormalities of the complexion. In one study, 46 percent of long-term smokers were found to have smoker's face.[8]

BLOOD

- Carbon monoxide—the colorless, odorless, deadly gas present in automobile exhaust—is present in cigarette smoke in more than 600 times the concentration considered safe in industrial plants. A smoker's blood typically contains 4 to 15 times as much carbon monoxide as that of a nonsmoker. This carbon monoxide stays in the bloodstream for up to six hours after you stop smoking. A 1982 University of Pittsburgh health survey found that nearly 80 percent of cigarette smokers had potentially hazardous levels of carbon monoxide in their blood. Research suggests that these abnormally high carbon monoxide levels may play a major role in triggering heart attacks.[9]

- When you breathe in a lungful of cigarette smoke, the carbon monoxide passes immediately into your blood, binding to the oxygen receptor sites and figuratively kicking the oxygen molecules out of your red blood cells. Hemoglobin that is bound to carbon monoxide is converted into carboxyhemoglobin, and is no longer able to transport oxygen. This means that less oxygen reaches a smoker's brain and other vital organs. Because of this added carbon monoxide load, a smoker's red cells are also less effective in removing carbon dioxide—a waste product—from his or her body's cells.

- If you continue to smoke for several weeks, your number of red cells begins to increase, as your body responds to chronic oxygen deprivation. This condition, characterized by an abnormally high level of red blood cells, is known as smoker's polycythemia. In addition, smoking makes your blood clot more easily. Both of these factors may increase your risk of heart attack or stroke.

MALE REPRODUCTIVE SYSTEM

- Two recent studies by Dr. Irving Goldstein and colleagues at the New England Male Reproductive Health Center, Boston University Medical School, found a possible link between smoking and erection problems. In the first study, the researchers found that among a population of 1,011 men with erection problems, 78 percent were smokers—more than twice the number of men with erection problems found in the general population. The researchers concluded that decreased potency might result from the negative effects of smoking on the blood vessels leading to the male reproductive organs.

- In their second study, the researchers measured the blood flow to the penis in 120 men who had come to their clinic with erection problems. They found that decrease in blood flow was proportional to the number of cigarettes smoked. Dr. Goldstein believes that smoking is the leading cause of impotence in the U.S. today.[10]

- In addition to diminishing potency, smoking adversely affects the fertility of male smokers by decreasing sperm count and sperm motility as well as altering sperm shape.[11]

FEMALE REPRODUCTIVE SYSTEM

- Women who smoke heavily show a 43 percent decline in fertility. Women smokers are three times more likely than nonsmokers to be infertile. Women who smoke also have fewer reproductive years: They reach menopause an average of 1¾ years earlier than nonsmokers.[12]

Smokers' Bodies Get Less Oxygen

Because carbon monoxide lowers your blood oxygen-carrying capacity, the blood delivers less oxygen to all the organs of the body. At the cellular level, oxygen is used to supply organs with the energy they need. Less oxygen means less energy.

In addition, more than thirty cancer-causing chemicals travel via the smoker's bloodstream to every organ of the body. The organs most sensitive to these carcinogens are the stomach, the kidneys, the bladder, and the cervix.

Cigarette smoking also weakens the immune system by depressing antibody response and depressing cell-mediated reactions to foreign invaders. As a result, smokers are more susceptible to a variety of infections.[13] These impairments are reversible if the smoker stops smoking.

Why Smoking Makes You Less Fit

Although a smoker's blood carries *less* oxygen, the nicotine in tobacco smoke increases the heart rate, requiring *more* oxygen. This is why smokers become short of breath more easily than nonsmokers. A group of researchers who tested the fitness levels of smokers and nonsmokers found that "Subjects with a smoking history showed a consistent impairment in performance at all stages of training when compared to subjects who had never smoked."[14] The high concentration of carbon monoxide also reduces the level of oxygen that is carried to the brain. This can produce lethargy, confusion, and difficulty in thinking clearly.

Smoking Impairs Taste and Smell

Continued smoking will also result in a loss of your senses of taste and smell. This occurs so gradually that it may go unnoticed, but the end result is the decreased sensitivity of two very important sense perceptions.

Smokers Die Younger

In addition to producing the short-term damage described above, smoking dramatically increases the risk of illness and death. Eight major studies, involving approximately 2 million people, have all found that smokers die sooner than nonsmokers. The average increase in death rate among smokers was 61 percent overall. For smokers in the two most vulnerable age groups—thirty-five to forty-five and forty-five to fifty-four—the death rates were 86 and 152 percent higher.[15]

A classic study by E.C. Hammond found that the average nonsmoker lives more than eight years longer than the average very heavy smoker.[16] Hammond's study looked at length of life in four classes of men: nonsmokers, light smokers (fewer than ten cigarettes per day), moderate smokers (10 to 19 cigarettes per day), heavy smokers (20 to 39 cigarettes per day), and very heavy smokers (40+ cigarettes per day). Assuming that each smoker began at age twenty-five, Hammond concluded that very heavy smokers, on average, died youngest, at age sixty-five. Heavy smokers were the next to die—at age sixty-seven. Moderate smokers lived a year longer—they died at age sixty-eight. Light smokers died at sixty-nine. But nonsmokers lived on to the ripe old age of seventy-three.

Thus, among the smokers in this study:

- *light* smokers gave up 4.6 years of life in exchange for smoking;
- *moderate* smokers gave up 5.5 years of life;
- *heavy* smokers gave up 6.2 years;
- *very heavy smokers* gave up 8.3 years.

These are average values, and are based on studies done while most men smoked unfiltered, high-tar cigarettes. It may well be that loss of life due to smoking is somewhat less for those who smoke filtered low-tar cigarettes.

Portion of U.S. Deaths Attributable to Smoking[35]	
lung cancer	85–90%
bronchitis & emphysema	85%
mouth cancers	70%
throat cancer	50%
bladder cancer	30–50%
esophagus cancer	20–40%
pancreas cancer	35%

arteriosclerosis	33%
heart disease	30%
kidney disease	15–25%

Smokers Have More Illnesses

In addition to dying younger, smokers have increased rates of both acute and chronic illnesses. The U.S. Public Health Service has estimated that cigarettes are responsible for:

- 81 million missed days of work per year;
- 145 million days spent ill in bed every year;
- 11 million additional cases of chronic illness per year;
- 280,000 additional cases of heart disease;
- 1 million additional cases of chronic bronchitis and emphysema;
- 1.8 million additional cases of chronic sinus problems;
- 1 million additional cases of peptic ulcer.

Compared to nonsmokers, smokers have higher rates of heart disease, emphysema, chronic bronchitis, peptic ulcer, allergies, and impairments of the immune system.[17] In addition, pregnant women who smoke have more stillbirths and babies of reduced birth weight. And children of smoking mothers are more likely to have continued difficulty developing physically, and even socially, throughout their lives. (The effects of smoking among pregnant women are discussed in detail in chapter 4.)

The harm done by tobacco smoke is dose-related: The more you smoke the higher the risk. Among continuing smokers, death rates are slightly lower for those who smoke low-tar cigarettes. The greatest possible improvement in health risk can be achieved by quitting tobacco altogether.

**Symptoms More Common in Smokers
than in Nonsmokers[34]**

Complaint	*Increase over nonsmokers*
cough	5.9×
shortness of breath	3.5×
easy fatigue	1.8×
insomnia	1.5×

LUNG AND OTHER CANCERS

Cancer is a term used to describe the abnormal growth of cells that may result in the destruction of healthy tissues. Persons exposed to certain environmental carcinogens are at increased risk of some cancers. Smokers who inhale tobacco smoke have been found to be at substantially increased risk for lung cancer. They are also at higher risk for cancers of the larynx, mouth, esophagus, bladder, kidney, and pancreas.

Smoking is the principal cause of the massive rise in death rates from lung cancer over the last forty years. The U.S. Public Health Service estimates that 85 to 90 percent of all U.S. lung cancers are caused by smoking.[18] The risk of lung cancer increases with the number of cigarettes smoked, the depth of inhalation, and the tar content of the cigarette.

The age at which smoking began is also a contributing factor in the development of lung cancer. Males who started smoking before the age of fifteen have nearly four times the rate of lung cancer as those who began smoking

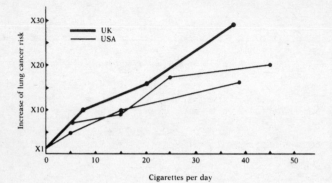

Figure 3–1 Relative Risk of Lung Cancer by Smoking Status Rates are for U.S. and U.K. male smokers and for Type I lung cancers.[20]

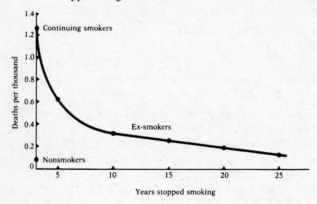

Figure 3–2 Decrease in Lung Cancer Risk for Ex-Smokers[21]

after age twenty-five. The cancer-producing effects of smoking are not seen for many years. It usually takes at least fifteen to twenty years of smoking to produce lung cancer in a human. *For those smokers who are able to quit, the risk of lung cancer begins to decrease immedi-*

ately. It continues to drop for the next ten to fifteen years, when it reaches a point only slightly higher than the risk for nonsmokers.[19]

CARDIOVASCULAR DISEASE

The effects of smoking on the heart and blood include increased blood clotting, an increased level of catecholamines, increased heart rate, decreased oxygen supply to the heart muscle, increased irritability of the electrical conducting system of the heart, and increased blood pressure. As a result, a smoker's risk of heart disease, stroke, and other vascular abnormalities is, on average, about twice that for nonsmokers.[22] The severity of heart attacks among smokers tends to be proportional to the cumulative dose of tobacco smoke they have inhaled in their entire smoking lives.[23]

A smoker's risk of heart disease may be increased substantially by the presence of other risk factors, as illustrated by Figure 3.3.

OTHER DISEASES AND CONDITIONS

- Emphysema—Virtually everyone with emphysema gets it as the result of smoking. Smokers are also at increased risk for chronic cough, respiratory infections, and audible abnormalities in the lungs.[25]

- Osteoporosis—Smokers are at increased risk of thinning of the bones. The bone fractures that result from loss of bone tissue are a major health problem, especially among postmenopausal women and both men and women over seventy. Researchers at the Mayo Clinic recently estimated that osteoporosis is responsible for 1.2 million fractures in the U.S. every year. Many of these fractures are fatal. Survivors frequently require long term nursing home care.[26]

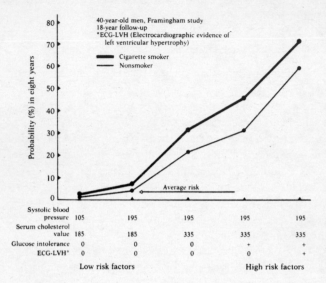

Figure 3-3 Risk of Heart Disease for Smokers with Other Risk Factors[24]

- Smokers experience more respiratory complications during surgery.

- A recent National Cancer Institute study showed that women who smoke have a one-and-one-half-fold risk of invasive cervical cancer. Women who smoke 40 or more cigarettes per day had a two-fold risk. Those who smoke unfiltered cigarettes are at particularly high risk.[27]

- Smokers are at increased risk of cancers of the larynx, mouth, esophagus, bladder, pancreas, kidney, and stomach.[28]

- Smokers are at increased risk for both peptic and duodenal ulcers.[29]

- Smokers are at increased risk of gum disease.[30]

- Recent studies suggest that smokers may be at fourfold risk of developing Alzheimer's disease.[31]

- Smokers are at increased risk of being hurt or killed in house fires—as are people who live with or near them. Thirty-nine percent of the people killed in fires caused by negligent use of cigarettes were *not* the smokers involved.[32]

Effects of Tobacco Smoke on Nonsmokers

Nonsmokers exposed to smoke-filled rooms show carbon monoxide blood levels equivalent to those of light smokers. Among adults exposed to tobacco smoke, the most common symptoms are eye irritation (reported by 69 percent of those who reported symptoms), headaches (33 percent), nasal irritation (33 percent), and cough (33 percent). Exposure to smoke can also trigger or aggravate allergic symptoms. Respiratory illness is more common in children exposed to tobacco smoke. And there is now considerable evidence to suggest that passive smoking may increase the risk of both heart attacks and lung cancer among the nonsmokers.[33]

Effects of Cutting Down and Quitting

The good news for smokers is that the great majority of negative health effects caused by smoking are *dose-related*. That is to say, the risk is proportional to the number of harmful particles that pass into the body. Thus every step you can take to reduce your "dose" of tobacco smoke will help improve your health. Quitting will reduce your risk the most, but cutting down can help reduce your risk as well. Strategies for cutting your smoking risk are discussed in chapters 4 through 7; strategies for quitting are discussed in chapters 8 through 12.

Harmful Substances in Cigarette Smoke

About 4,000 chemical compounds are produced when tobacco burns. The following constituents of cigarette smoke are known or suspected to be harmful to the human body:[37]

acetaldehyde
acetone
acetonitrile
acrolein
acrylonitrile
alcohols
ammonia
amphenols
arsenic
benza(a)anthracene
benzene
benzo(a)pyrene
benzo(j)fluoranthene
benzo(g,h,i)perylene
butylamine
cadmium compounds
carbon dioxide
carbon monoxide
catechol
creols
DDT
dibenz(a,j)acridine
dibenz(a,h)acridine
dibenzo(c,g)carbazole
diethylnitrosamine
dimethylamine
dimethylnitrosamine
endrin
ethylmethylnitrosamine
fluoranthene
formaldehyde
furfural
hydrazine
hydrocyanic acid

hydrogen cyanide
naphthalenes
nickel compounds
nicotine
nitric oxide
nitriles
nitrogen oxides
N-nitrosonornicotine
nitrosopyrrolidine
polonium-210
pyrene
vinyl chloride

• • •

1-methylindoles
3- & 4-methylcatechols
5-methylchrysene
9-methylcarbazoles

• • •

other acids
other catechols
other ketones
other metallic ions
other nitrogen-containing
    compounds
other nitrosamines
other phenols
other polynuclear aromatic
    hydrocarbons
other radioactive com-
    pounds
other sulfur-containing
    compounds

4

Are You a High- or Low-Risk Smoker?

Because of the way newspapers, radio, and TV deal with risk, it's difficult for us to understand the relative importance of the various risks in our lives. We read newspaper headlines about products that have been taken off the market because consuming them might lead to a one-in-a-million chance of getting cancer. Many smokers quite understandably feel that if cigarettes *really* posed a substantial health risk, they would hear more about it than they presently do. Unfortunately, this is not the case.

1,475 Deaths Per Day

If three commercial 747 jumbo jets were to crash every day for an entire year, it would certainly make front-page news. And deservedly so, for this would add up to about *540,000 deaths per year*. But according to one current estimate, the number of premature deaths caused or accelerated by cigarette smoking works out to the same number.[1] This adds up to *1,475 deaths per day*. Other experts have estimated the number of excess deaths at 350,000 per year, "merely" 1,000 excess deaths per day.[2]

If you knew that three jumbo jets would go down in flames today, you would probably be extremely wary about boarding a commercial airliner. Yet 54 million smokers light up every day, most of them without a second thought.

What Makes a "Tragedy"?

The risk of dying in a plane crash and the risk of smoking-related disease are treated quite differently for a number of reasons:

Unexpected, surprising news triggers terror and fear, while the "same old story" has lost its news value and is easily ignored. Furthermore, when misfortune befalls a large group of people together, it is perceived as much more "tragic" than if the same number of individuals were to suffer a similar fate individually. Thus, if a bus containing sixty people is involved in a traffic accident and all occupants are killed, this is considered a much more important "tragedy" than if sixty motorists were to die in sixty separate accidents.

Voluntary vs. Involuntary Risks

In addition to the factors above, people will accept risks that are substantially higher—as much as 100 times higher—*if they are able to choose such activities freely*. People don't like to be forced to accept risks—even though they might choose to take similar or greater risks in other matters. This helps explain the unwillingness of nonsmokers to accept even the relatively small risks of "passive" smoking—because they are forced to breathe tobacco smoke against their will.

As Urquhart and Heilmann write, "People will engage in fairly hair-raising activities on their own initiative, while steadfastly maintaining their right to protest vehemently when forced into something quite tame by comparison."[3] And when a risk is accepted by a sizable proportion of the population, as it is in the case of smoking, it is much easier for an individual to accept it.

Some smokers console themselves that although smoking may indeed be dangerous, they could just as easily be murdered on the street or die in an auto accident. But a review of the facts makes it clear that this is little more than a convenient self-deception. As one researcher wrote, "Of every 1,000 young male smokers, one will be murdered, six will die on the roads, and 250 will be killed by tobacco-related diseases."[4]

Average Risks vs. Actual Risks

The smoking-related risks of heart disease, cancer, and other diseases are discussed in the previous chapter. But these are all average risks. Some smokers are at even higher risk of being injured or killed by smoking. You may be at increased risk if:

- you have a medical condition that is made worse by smoking;
- you have an inherited susceptibility to a smoking-related disease;
- you are exposed to environmental or occupational toxins;
- you are an especially heavy smoker;
- psychological or social factors might make it especially difficult for you to quit, even if you should decide to do so.

Risk Is Proportional to Total Lifetime Dose

When a physician or other health professional takes a complete medical history, one item that is always included, for smokers, is the Total Lifetime Dose (TLD) of tobacco smoke. The TLD, usually expressed in pack-years, is a rough approximation of the number of cigarettes you have consumed over your lifetime. One pack-year equals 365 packs or 7,300 cigarettes. Since patterns of inhalation vary widely from smoker to smoker, a pack-year is a relatively rough measure.

Two smokers' actual effective dose of tar, carbon monoxide, and nicotine may vary considerably, even though they may have smoked the same number of cigarettes over their lifetime:

- Those who smoke low-tar brands may be exposed to less tar (though not necessarily less carbon monoxide) than those who smoke unfiltered, high-tar brands.

- Those who take more puffs per cigarette are at greater risk than those who take fewer puffs.

- Those who smoke their cigarette farther down, leaving shorter butts, are at greater risk than those who extinguish their cigarette earlier.

- Those who inhale deeply are at greater risk than those who inhale little or no smoke.

With these qualifications, the factor that seems to be proportional to risk is your total lifetime dose (TLD)— the total number of cigarettes you have smoked since your very first cigarette.

Calculating Your Lifetime Dose

Your total lifetime dose is proportional to the average number of cigarettes smoked per day times the number of years you have smoked. This number is relatively easy to calculate:

1. Determine the number of years you have smoked.
2. Determine the approximate number of packs you smoked per day for each year.
3. Add up the pack-year figures to get your lifetime smoking dose.

Here's an example:

Maria Taylor began smoking in 1961, at age seventeen. She smoked approximately a half pack per day until 1968, when she got married. She then began smoking about a pack a day. This continued until 1975, when she took a stressful job, and began smoking two packs a day. In 1981 she changed jobs and cut back to a pack a day. She remained at that level through 1987.

Dates	Years	Packs per day	Pack-years
1961–1968	8	½	4
1969–1975	7	1	7
1976–1981	6	2	12
1982–1988	7	1	7

Total Lifetime Dose   30   pack-years

Duplicate the form below on a separate sheet of paper and use it to calculate your own Total Lifetime Dose.

Dates	Years	Packs per day	Pack-years
_____	___	_____	_____
_____	___	_____	_____
_____	___	_____	_____
_____	___	_____	_____
_____	___	_____	_____

Total Lifetime Dose _____ pack-years

Your health risk is roughly proportional to your total lifetime dose. The greater your lifetime dose, the greater your risk of coming down with a smoking-related disease. Thus, if you have smoked three packs a day for fifty years, you would have a TLD of 150. If you have smoked ten cigarettes per day for four years, you would have a TLD of 2.

Ten Types of High-Risk Smokers

The sections that follow outline ten risk factors that can make some individuals more vulnerable to smoking-related injury or disease. These high-risk categories are as follows:

1. Pregnant women.
2. Women over thirty who take birth control pills.
3. Members of families at high risk for heart disease.
4. Smokers who already have smoking-related diseases.
5. Smokers exposed to toxic agents in the workplace.
6. Smokers with high-risk lifestyles.
7. Smokers with high-risk personalities.

8. Smokers about to undergo surgery.
9. Smokers with abnormal lab tests or family histories.
10. Smokers who are heavily addicted to nicotine.

1. PREGNANT WOMEN

The babies of women who smoke suffer from a variety of negative consequences, including lower birth weight, shorter stature, smaller head and arm circumferences, higher risk of prematurity, higher risk of spontaneous abortion, decreased fetal movements, increased risk of early rupture of fetal membranes, and higher risk of neurological impairment when compared to the babies of nonsmokers. The decrease in birth weight is greatest if the mother is a heavy smoker. Maternal smoking has negative effects on the baby's breathing; moreover, the baby's heart rate increases as soon as its mother lights up a cigarette. Overall, the risk of death during or before birth is 27 percent higher for the babies of smoking mothers.

Researchers believe that smoking slows the baby's growth through two independent pathways:

- Carbon monoxide poisoning—Carbon monoxide passes freely from the mother's circulatory system into the baby's bloodstream and tissues, decreasing the baby's available oxygen levels.

- Increased catecholamine levels—Nicotine increases the release of catecholamines, hormones that narrow the baby's arteries and limit blood flow.

Most researchers would now agree that prospective mothers who smoke during pregnancy may well be committing inadvertent child abuse. *If there is one group of smokers who should most definitely quit smoking, it is pregnant women.*

If all efforts at quitting fail, pregnant women should, at the very least, (1) reduce their smoking to five or less low-tar cigarettes per day, and (2) supplement their diet with extra portions of milk, eggs, and cheese during their pregnancy. For a detailed description of the effects of food supplements on the birth weight of babies whose mothers smoked during pregnancy, see the journal article by Jack Metcoff et al.[5] (You may order a copy of this article for $2.00 postpaid from the Center for Self-Care Studies, 3805 Stevenson Avenue, Austin, Texas 78703.)

It is now well established that reduction of smoking during pregnancy improves the birth weight of the infant. Quitting smoking altogether during pregnancy provides optimal conditions for fetal growth.[6]

2. WOMEN OVER THIRTY WHO TAKE BIRTH CONTROL PILLS

Since 1978, all birth control pills have carried the following warning: "Cigarette smoking increases the risk of serious cardiovascular side effects from oral contraceptive use." The most dangerous side effects are heart attack and stroke. Risks are particularly high for smokers over thirty and *extraordinarily* high for smokers over forty. Here is a table of risk of death for the following classes of women:

Risk of Death for Women Using the Pill
(Rates per 100,000 users per year)

Age	Nonsmokers	Smokers
25–29	1.2	1.4
30–34	1.8	10.4
35–39	3.9	12.8
40–44	6.6	58.4

The risks are higher for women who smoke more than 25 cigarettes per day. Women under thirty-five can take the Pill without increasing their risk to dangerous levels *provided they do not smoke*. Women over forty who do not smoke should take the Pill only in extreme situations. Smokers over thirty who are on the Pill and are unable to quit should switch to another form of birth control.[7]

3. MEMBERS OF FAMILIES AT HIGH RISK FOR HEART DISEASE

Have any of your close relatives died of heart disease before age forty-five? If they have, and you smoke, you have three times the normal risk of developing smoking-related heart disease. Studies done at the University of Utah School of Medicine suggest that such people may have a genetic susceptibility to early coronary disease. This hypothesis was borne out by a British study in which researchers found that the children of heart attack victims had lower levels of high-density lipoprotein (HDL), a "good" form of cholesterol.[8]

4. SMOKERS WHO ALREADY HAVE SMOKING-RELATED DISEASES

Such diseases include heart disease, lung cancer, emphysema, chronic bronchitis, ulcers, high blood pressure, diabetes, osteoporosis, blood clots in the legs, and glaucoma.[9]

- Heart disease—One study that looked at the effects of quitting among smokers who had experienced unstable angina or a previous heart attack found that 82 percent of those who continued to smoke died over the thirteen years the study was in progress. Of smokers who quit, only 37 percent died during that period.

- Ulcers—Untreated ulcer patients are 3.4 times as likely to experience recurrent ulcer symptoms if they smoke. And the harmful effects of smoking more than counteract the benefits of treatment with the most widely used antiulcer drug (cimetidine). Studies show that among ulcer patients, untreated nonsmokers experience fewer symptoms than smokers who received treatment.

- High Blood Pressure—Smoking increases blood pressure and is one of the fundamental risk factors for high blood pressure. Furthermore, persons with high blood pressure who smoke regularly are more likely to develop the accelerated form of the disease than those who do not smoke. Smoking can also interfere with effective medical therapy for high blood pressure: The average heavy smoker has a blood pressure 10 to 15 points higher than the average nonsmoker.

- Diabetes—Diabetics who smoke are approximately eight times more likely to complicate their disease than nonsmoking diabetics. Smoking increases the likelihood of arterial blockages in the legs, a common symptom in diabetics. And diabetic smokers are twice as likely to develop arteriosclerosis.

- Osteoporosis—Women with osteoporosis (particularly those who are slender) seem to be at increased risk of bone thinning if they smoke. Smoking apparently increases the rate of breakdown of estrogen, which helps protect women against osteoporosis. Slender women are apparently at increased risk because fat cells produce a small quantity of estrogen. In addition, women with osteoporosis are much more likely to lose their teeth if they smoke. One study of women with osteoporosis found that smokers were three times as likely to lose their teeth during their fifties as nonsmokers.

Osteoporosis is one of the most underpublicized diseases of our times. This condition is responsible for 1.2 million fractures per year in elderly women and men.

• Glaucoma—Persons who smoke are at increased risk of getting or aggravating glaucoma, since smoking increases intraocular pressure.

5. SMOKERS EXPOSED TO TOXIC AGENTS IN THE WORKPLACE

No chemical or industrial by-product comes close to equaling tobacco smoke as a health hazard. One group of researchers estimates that smoking 1.4 cigarettes produces a risk of loss of life comparable to consuming 100 charcoal-broiled steaks or living near to a polyvinyl-chloride (PVC) plant for twenty years. The categories of workers listed below may be exposed to toxic substances that combine with tobacco smoke to put smokers at a significantly greater risk than nonsmokers exposed to these same substances:

• Workers exposed to carbon monoxide (firefighters, traffic control officers, traffic police, bus drivers, tunnel workers, and turnpike workers).

• Workers exposed to asbestos. Asbestos workers who smoke may be at fifty-fold risk of lung disease compared to nonsmokers not exposed to asbestos.

• Workers exposed to sulfur dioxide, uranium, coal and coal dust, cotton dust, mineral dusts, and other particulate matter (silica, mica, iron oxide, aluminum oxide) show small airway damage similar to that suffered by asbestos workers. Thus, they may be at similar risk for lung disease.

• Quarry workers, mine workers, grain workers, forestry

workers, woodworkers, construction workers, iron and
steel foundry workers, aluminum workers, shipyard
workers, workers in the motor vehicle industry, rubber
workers, hospital workers exposed to high levels of
ethylene oxide (a chemical used to sterilize surgical
instruments).

- Workers exposed to arsenic, beryllium, chloromethyl
ethers, chromium, radiation, mustard gas, or nickel,
and those who worked in factories manufacturing polyvinylchloride before 1975.[10]

6. SMOKERS WITH HIGH-RISK LIFESTYLES

Current research suggests that the following groups of
smokers are at increased risk from smoking and/or are
much more likely to smoke.

- People who are overweight—especially those with substantial fat deposits in their abdomens. Swedish researchers have found that people with an abdominal fat
pattern (in plain language, a big belly) are at increased
risk for both heart attack and stroke. Here's the easiest
way to determine whether you have this pattern: Take
your waist and hip measurements, then divide your
waist measurement by your hip measurement. A ratio
of more than 1.0 in men or 0.8 in women suggests that
you may be at increased risk.[11]

- People who are extremely thin—some studies suggest
that people who are underweight are more likely to be
smokers.[12]

- Heavy drinkers—studies show that cigarette smoking is
much more common among those who are regular
heavy drinkers. And smokers take deeper puffs when
they drink alcohol. In addition, heavy alcohol use en-
hances the cancer-causing effects of tobacco smoke.

Heavy drinkers who also smoke heavily have 6 to 15 times the risk of oral cancers and of cancers of the larynx and esophagus, compared to nonsmoking non-drinkers.[13]

- People who are unmarried, divorced, or separated—Studies show that smoking is more common among these groups.[14]

- Lack of exercise—Lack of exercise contributes to heart diseases. Smoking coupled with a weight problem makes the risk considerably worse.

7. SMOKERS WITH HIGH-RISK PERSONALITIES

Research by the Department of Health and Human Services shows that, on average, smokers' personalities differ from those of nonsmokers. Smokers tend to be more extroverted, defiant, and impulsive. They are more likely to take risks and more likely to be divorced or separated. They consume more alcohol, coffee, psychoactive drugs, and aspirin than nonsmokers.[15] Researchers have suggested several psychological factors that may make people high-risk smokers:

- Preference for high-risk activities—Some studies suggest that smoking is more frequent among people who enjoy risk-taking behavior. Some people may smoke in part because of an unusually strong urge to take risks.[16]

- Predisposition to being accident-prone—Some studies show that smokers are more likely to have accidents and are less likely to take measures to reduce risks, e.g., wearing seat belts.[17]

- Type A personality—Many studies of the psychological basis of heart disease suggest that there is a high-risk personality that is at increased risk for heart disease. These so-called Type A people tend to "blow up" over minor irritants, getting angrier than the situation really calls for. Though there's usually a reason for these outbursts—a driver who pulls in front of you in traffic, finding yourself on a long line at the bank—these minor disturbances merely serve as triggers for a preexisting reservoir of hostility. As a person's Type A behavior becomes more extreme, these outbursts may be triggered by events of an even more trivial nature.

The Type A hypothesis, originally proposed by San Francisco cardiologists Meyer Friedman and Ray Rosenman, has become widely accepted as a risk factor for heart disease. Friedman identifies an aspect of this condition, this increased urgency about the passage of time, as "hurry sickness." He believes that this harmful tendency affects more than half of all professional and executive American men, as well a growing number of women.

Friedman believes that Type A people drive themselves ceaselessly and senselessly because they suffer from a hidden lack of self-esteem. This yearning for self-esteem is so intense that it drives them into a state of hyperaggressiveness—a state in which they may feel indifferent to the feelings or fundamental rights of their coworkers, competitors, or opponents.

Friedman and his colleagues have recently completed a study that demonstrates that the Type A behavior pattern can be modified. The best antidote is to slow down, to learn to relax, to polish the skills of friendship, to learn to seek out pleasure, to see the wonder and adventure in other people—not merely to see them as means to your own ends. (For more on modifying Type A behavior, see chapter 5.)[18]

8. SMOKERS ABOUT TO UNDERGO SURGERY

Studies show that complications during surgery are as much as 2.4 times higher in smokers. This effect can be considerably reversed by a mere twelve hours without cigarettes. The principal culprit is carbon monoxide. Smoking reduces the oxygen-carrying capacity of your blood; this is especially dangerous during anesthesia.[19]

9. SMOKERS WITH ABNORMAL LAB TESTS OR FAMILY HISTORIES

The following risk factors may significantly increase your smoking risks:

- A family history of high blood pressure—If your parents, grandparents, brothers, or sisters had or have high blood pressure, you may be at increased risk of developing heart disease as the result of your smoking.[20]

- High serum cholesterol—People with high serum cholesterol levels are at increased risk of heart disease.[21]

Risk	Total Cholesterol
Very low risk (½ average risk)	150 or less
Low risk	200
Average risk	225
Moderate Risk (2 × normal)	260
High risk (3 × normal)	300 and above

- Emphysema—If a close family member smoked and had emphysema, you may be at increased risk of emphysema if you smoke. An inherited deficiency of certain lung enzymes can produce increased vulnerability to smoke-caused injuries that lead to emphysema.[22]

- High heart rate—Death rates from heart disease, as well

as a number of other conditions, are higher for people who have higher pulse rates.[23]

- Abnormal EKG (also called ECG, electrocardiograph). Studies show that smokers with major EKG abnormalities have higher death rates.[24]

- High hematocrit—A Puerto Rican study suggests that middle-aged men with a higher hematocrit (more than 49 percent) had a significantly higher risk of heart disease, heart attack, and heart-disease related death than those whose hematocrit was lower (less than 42 percent). The hematocrit measures the percentage of blood volume that is made up of red blood cells.[25]

Normal hematocrit values are as follows:

Men:	40–54%
Women:	37–47%

10. SMOKERS WHO ARE HEAVILY ADDICTED TO NICOTINE

Persons who are strongly addicted to nicotine are usually heavier smokers and tend to have a more difficult time cutting down or quitting because of their extreme degree of nicotine dependence. One key sign of being heavily addicted is needing a cigarette immediately after awakening. The number of minutes between waking and lighting the first cigarette of the day appears to be a useful index of addiction. One heavy smoker we interviewed explained that he kept an open pack next to his alarm clock so he could switch off the alarm and reach for his cigarettes in a single gesture.

Other signs of intense addiction include:

- Experiencing the first cigarette of the day as the most satisfying.

- Smoking heavily first thing in the morning.
- Having difficulty refraining from smoking in no-smoking areas.
- Smoking more than 25 cigarettes per day.
- Being unable to cut down or quit even when you are ill.
- Smoking high-nicotine or unfiltered cigarettes.
- Inhaling deeply on every puff.
- Smoking each cigarette down to a short butt.
- Lighting a new cigarette immediately after finishing the last one.
- Experiencing severe anxiety about running out of cigarettes.[26]

What To Do If You're a High-Risk Smoker

Smokers who fall into one or more of the high-risk groups listed above may be especially interested in the risk reduction strategies described in chapters 5 through 12. Heavily addicted smokers should explore the possibility of switching to less harmful sources of nicotine. (See chapter 9.)

Getting
Ready
to Quit

5 ～⚬⚬

Exercise, Eating, Stress Skills, and Social Support for Smokers

In addition to making some of the changes in specific smoking behaviors described elsewhere in *The No-Nag, No-Guilt, Do-It-Your-Own-Way Guide to Quitting Smoking*, health-concerned smokers may wish to take advantage of the benefits of some general lifestyle changes. Adopting healthier ways of eating, exercising, managing stress, and getting support from friends and family are changes that would benefit anyone, whether they smoke or not.

Adopting such general pro-health measures can be a valuable first step for smokers who don't feel ready to make a firm commitment to quitting. These approaches can help you decrease your overall health risk while you build a solid foundation for quitting.

A healthier lifestyle is a no-lose proposition. Although there is as yet only a moderate amount of evidence on the direct risk reduction effects of such lifestyle changes for smokers, the evidence we *do* have is most encouraging. Even more encouraging is the evidence that these lifestyle measures—especially exercise—can greatly in-

65

crease your chances of cutting down and can increase
your chances of eliminating smoking altogether.

I. EXERCISE

Exercise provides many of the same rewards as
smoking—mental sharpening, an increased sense of control, and a greater ability to relax. Many successful ex-
smokers have found that they were able to reduce or
eliminate smoking only after they started a regular exercise program. Exercise plays an important part in many
professionally-run smoking control programs. "In treating hundreds of smokers, I saw that the ones who partic-
ipated in aerobic exercise were most likely to quit," says
psychologist Olvide Pomerleau, director of the behavioral medicine program at the University of Michigan
School of Medicine.[1]

A recent Gallup Poll showed that people who exercise
regularly were twice as likely to quit smoking as nonex-
ercisers.[2] As Dr. John Kaufman recently wrote in the
New England Journal of Medicine, "[Anti-smoking programs based on aerobic exercise] have had high success
rates in motivating smokers to quit. One of the best types
of aerobic exercise is a running-jogging program. . . .
The runner finds that he is unable to run and smoke because of marked discomfort at running anything but short
distances."[3] An Ohio State University study found that
following a regular exercise program helped many smokers quit. Those who didn't quit reduced their smoking
level substantially.[4]

A study published in the journal *Preventive Medicine*
found that men who voluntarily increased their fitness
level were significantly more likely to cut down or quit

than those who maintained a more sedentary lifestyle.[5] And Stanford University's Dr. Peter Wood calls exercise "the all-purpose risk reducer."[6]

There seem to be several reasons for the beneficial effects of exercise on smokers' addiction:

- Regular physical activity induces biochemical changes within the body. Some of these changes are similar to those produced by nicotine. Exercise boosts catecholamines, producing increased mental alertness. And sustained exercise increases the brain's production of endorphins, which produce euphoria and a pleasant, relaxed feeling.

- The act of working regular exercise into your daily schedule helps provide a regular "island of peace" that can interrupt the smoker's chronic stress cycles.

- Regular gentle exercise tones smokers' muscles and helps them feel more relaxed.

- Regular exercise helps people cope more effectively with the daily hassles of modern life. It also decreases feelings of anxiety and depression. In addition, exercise produces more restful sleep, which in turn helps the exerciser stay calm and deal more effectively with stress.

- Regular exercise can produce positive personality changes. As one team of researchers reported: "When a sedentary, middle-aged man decides to enter a long-term, strenuous physical conditioning program and disciplines himself to stick it out, he will often gain a sense of accomplishment, independence, and sense of control over his own life that he never had before. He is also likely to become more resolute, emotionally stable and imaginative, and this is an exhilarating experience.[7]

Here are some of the benefits of regular exercise reported by subjects in one such study:[8]

Exercise Program Effects	Subjects Reporting Benefit
Increased stamina	90%
Feelings of better health	85%
Weight reduction	67%
Improved work performance	60%
Decreased food intake	48%
Increased recreation	45%
Reduced stress and tension	43%
More positive work attitude	40%
Better sleep	37%

Can Exercise Lower Smokers' Health Risks?

In addition to these psychological benefits, a few studies suggest that smokers who begin exercising regularly may also obtain some small degree of protection against the health risks of smoking.

A 1986 study of nearly 17,000 Harvard alumni showed that *among men who smoked more than a pack of cigarettes per day, those who exercised regularly had 30 percent lower death rates*. Regular physical activity also decreased death rates among those with high blood pressure and those with inherited tendencies toward early death. The researchers concluded that for smokers and nonsmokers alike, regular moderate exercise seems to be "the key to longevity."[9]

A study by E. Cuyler Hammond compared the effects of exercise on both smokers and nonsmokers:

**Exercise, Smoking, and Relative Risk of Death
from Heart Disease**[10]

Exercise Level	Never Smoked	Smoked a Pack or More Per Day
No exercise	1.8	3.0
Slight exercise	1.2	2.8
Moderate exercise	1.0	2.3
Heavy exercise	1.0	2.1

This study too suggests that death rates for smokers who exercise are somewhat lower than the death rates for smokers who do not exercise.

But many medical experts believe that it is a disservice to suggest that exercise can offer any added protection for smokers. According to Dr. Kenneth H. Cooper, president of the Aerobics Center in Dallas and author of *The Aerobics Program for Total Well-Being* and *Running Without Fear*: "Contrary to what many smokers would like to believe, exercise can't counteract the damage being done to your body while you continue to smoke. What exercise can do is help you kick the habit. . . . I have received hundreds of letters from cigarette smokers telling me how they could never break the habit until they started exercising. Regular aerobic activity seems to have given them an overall discipline and self-confidence they didn't have before."[11]

Thus the question of whether exercise offers protective effects for continuing smokers remains controversial, but there is widespread agreement that smokers who *do* begin exercising regularly receive a three-fold benefit from their exercise program:

- Exercise makes you feel better about yourself.
- Exercise helps you handle stress more effectively.

• Exercise makes it much easier to cut down or quit.

Exercise as a Positive Addiction

Some researchers have called exercise a positive addiction. Many physicians—including cardiologist and running guru George Sheehan—have suggested that starting an exercise program is the single most helpful thing a health-concerned smoker can do.

"I've never advised any of my patients to stop smoking," Sheehan says. "I've even, on occasion, advised a patient who'd quit to *start* smoking again—because he'd gained 15 pounds and was beating up on his kids. But when smokers start *exercising*, they frequently find themselves quitting without even *meaning* to. The need to smoke just seems to go away. The well-toned body has a mind of its own, and it will either stop smoking or will cut down to a level that's no longer in the danger area.

"Smokers who start exercising find that they can use exercise—rather than cigarettes—to deal with tension. Instead of taking ten and having a smoke, instead of counting to ten, I encourage my smoking patients to go out and *run* ten."[12]

Even weight lifting may help reduce your risk of heart disease. A recent study at the University of Oregon found that formerly sedentary men and women who went through a sixteen-week program of weight training showed substantially lower cholesterol levels.[13]

In addition, people who are physically unfit are more likely to develop high blood pressure. Starting a program of regular exercise before quitting can also help you keep your weight under control after you quit.

If you do your exercise in a situation in which there is also social support, such as in a group or with a friend, you may reap additional benefits from your exercise plan. Local jogging or walking groups can be good places to find an exercise buddy. Or you can arrange to go walking or jogging with a friend.

Starting an Exercise Program

Sheehan advises: "The best starting place for beginners is to find a way to get out and break a sweat every day." Kenneth Cooper recommends that you engage in gentle aerobic exercise for at least 30 minutes per session a minimum of three (ideally four or more) sessions per week.

Smokers who are in extremely poor shape, those who have medical problems, and those over thirty-five who have not exercised in many years, should either consult a physician or read Cooper's excellent book, *Running Without Fear: How to Reduce the Risk of Heart Attack and Sudden Death During Aerobic Exercise*, before starting an exercise program. (Cooper's title is somewhat misleading—the book covers all kinds of exercise, not just running.)

Choosing Your Exercise(s)

What type of exercise is best for you? The exercise you enjoy the most and find most convenient. Here's a self-scored quiz that can help you choose one or more types of exercise that might fit most easily into your life. A list of possible exercises is given below. The starred items have the most pronounced aerobic training effect.

Pick the *five* types of exercise that seem most appealing and practical, then use a separate piece of paper to rate each of your five choices on a scale

of 1 to 10 for both *appeal* and *convenience*. Add
the two scores for each exercise to get your total.

*Walking	*Aerobic dance
*Jogging or running	Gardening
*Swimming	Golf
*Exercise bike (stationary)	Tennis
*Outdoor bicycling	Racquetball
*Cross-country skiing	Handball
*Rowing machine	Volleyball
*Jumping rope	Calisthenics
*Running in place	Weight training

Michael P., one of the health-concerned smokers we
interviewed, had always felt that he "should" start a regular jogging program. Yet somehow he had never gotten
around to it. When he took this quiz, he realized that he
really *dreaded* the idea of running. He was delighted to
find that there were several *other* kinds of exercise that
suited him nicely. This is how he completed the quiz:

Activity	Convenient	Desirable	Total
Walking	10	8	18
Tennis	6	10	16
Gardening	8	4	12
Outdoor bicycling	4	6	10
Jogging	7	2	9

Many smokers find that walking is a good exercise to
start with. It can be done anywhere and requires no special equipment other than a comfortable pair of walking
shoes. Several of the successful quitters we interviewed
said that they had used walking to help them quit. They
recommend starting out by taking brief, brisk walks during the times of day when you are accustomed to doing
your heaviest smoking.

In addition to regular exercise periods, you can take exercise "minibreaks" whenever you feel the urge for a cigarette: Take a quick walk around the block. Do a quick stretch or a few push-ups. One of our interview subjects told us that when she had an urge for a cigarette she would go into the bathroom and jog in place for three minutes.

The First Three Months

It usually takes about three months—roughly a hundred days—for an exercise program to become a regular part of your life. During this time, do everything you can to make it easy for you to exercise: Schedule exercise times on your calendar. Find a regular exercise buddy. Make appointments to exercise with friends. Ask your spouse to support your efforts—this is vitally important in maintaining an exercise program. Make a pact with yourself that you'll continue exercising for one hundred days, then reassess your exercise program. At the end of that time, chances are it will be an old and valued part of your daily routine.

II. EATING

Some researchers believe that unhealthy eating habits may be responsible for nearly as many deaths as smoking. The harmful effects of a high-fat diet in heart disease are well known, and the Center for Science in the Public Interest estimates that diet plays a key role in more than 133,000 cancer deaths per year in the U.S. Researchers estimate that diet is responsible for 30 to 40 percent of all cancers in men and 60 percent of all cancers in women. A recent report by the National Cancer Institute suggests the following guidelines to help reduce your cancer risk:[14]

1. Eat less fat.
2. Eat more fruits, vegetables, and whole grains.
3. Eat fewer foods that are smoked, pickled, or cured.
4. Avoid food additives.
5. If you drink, do so in moderation.

Valuable Vegetables

There is substantial evidence to suggest that a high-vegetable diet can be especially beneficial. A Japanese study of 122,000 men over forty suggests that eating vegetables every day can substantially reduce a person's risk of getting cancer. Researchers estimated that such other life-style factors as eating red meat and drinking alcohol may also increase one's cancer risk. Subjects who smoked, ate red meat, and drank alcohol but did not eat vegetables daily were 2.5 times as likely to die of cancer as those who ate vegetables daily but did not drink, smoke, or eat red meat. The researchers estimated that *even heavy smokers can reduce their chances of dying of cancer by eating more vegetables*. Dr. Takeshi Hirayama speculates that this protective effect may be due to the vitamin A, vitamin C, fiber, and other nutrients in vegetables.[15]

This Japanese study backs up the U.S. National Cancer Institute's campaign to persuade the U.S. population to eat more fruits and vegetables while cutting back on fat. The recommendations of the NCI, as well as those of many other nutrition experts, can be summed up in this simple jingle:

Eat more vegies,
Eat less fat.
Greens and grains
Are where it's at.[16]

And Don't Forget Fruit

A recent study by the American Cancer Society suggests that eating fruit or drinking fruit juice regularly may "somewhat reduce the high risk of lung cancer incurred by cigarette smoking." The study examined the dietary habits of one million male smokers. The researchers found that as the amount of fruit a person consumed went up, their cancer risk went down. *Lung cancer rates for smokers who consumed fruit or fruit juice five to seven times per week were 44 percent lower than for smokers who consumed fruit twice a week or less.*[17]

The body's defenses—against cancer and other diseases—require certain nutrients to function effectively. Present studies suggest that in addition to vegetables, fruits, and grains, the most important anticancer nutrients are vitamins A, C, and E, selenium, isothiocyanates, indoles, calcium, and fiber. And of all the cancer-*promoting* nutrients, the most important are probably fat, alcohol, and food additives.[18]

Vitamin A

Vitamin A is probably the single most important nutrient for healthy maintenance of the tissues lining the bronchi, trachea, and lungs. If you are deficient in vitamin A, the cilia that normally cleanse the lungs and bronchial passages are more susceptible to injury by tobacco smoke and the goblet cells, which secrete mucus, are more likely to die.

Vitamin A protects laboratory animals from carcinogenic substances found in cigarette smoke. Hamsters exposed to a carcinogen resisted cancer more effectively if they had been given vitamin A supplements. In addition, vitamin A can help prevent cancers of the skin, bladder, and breast in laboratory animals.

There is substantial evidence that vitamin A may be equally effective in protecting human smokers. Vitamin A is broken down at a faster rate in smokers, probably because some of the substances in tobacco smoke inactivate this vitamin. Several studies have shown that persons with low blood levels of vitamin A are more likely to come down with cancer. One study showed that heavy long-term smokers who were given a six-month course of vitamin A showed a decreased level of precancerous changes in their bronchi. And while the results of some studies have been less conclusive, a Norwegian study found that heavy smokers with low vitamin A levels had three times as much cancer as heavy smokers who had adequate blood levels of vitamin A. A number of studies suggest that vitamin A may also have a protective effect against cervical cancer.

The American Cancer Society now recommends a diet high in vitamin A to help prevent cancer. Michael B. Sporn, chief of the lung cancer branch in the Division of Cancer Cause and Prevention at the National Cancer Institute, has stated that ''No human population at risk for development of cancer should be allowed to remain in a vitamin A deficient state. Considering the relatively trivial cost . . . this is certainly a goal which should be met for the entire population.''[19]

Vitamin researcher Sheldon Saul Hendler, in reviewing the studies done on vitamin A's role in protecting smokers, concludes that there is a good deal of evidence to suggest that vitamin A may, in fact, protect against some of the ravages of smoking. But he warns that smokers should *not* interpret this to mean that if they take vitamin A, they can go on smoking without risk. Such protection would, at best, be only partial.[20]

Vitamin A is available in two forms, fully formed vitamin A (technically known as *retinol*), and several pre-vitamin A substances, most notably *beta-carotene*, which are converted to vitamin A inside the body. Preformed vitamin A can have toxic effects at relatively low levels, but beta-carotene is relatively nontoxic because it is converted into the active form very slowly.

Beta-carotene is found in dark yellow, orange, and green fruits and vegetables such as carrots, broccoli, asparagus, apricots, and cantaloupe. One simple way to increase the level of vitamin A in your diet is to add carrots to your snacking menu. My friend and colleague Joe Graedon, author (with Teresa Graedon) of *The People's Pharmacy*, dutifully crunches his way through three carrots a day. He suggests that smokers—and nonsmokers as well—would be well advised to do likewise.[21]

Vitamin C

Vitamin C, also known as ascorbic acid, is an active antioxidant, and can block the formation of some cancer-causing substances, especially the nitrosamines. These carcinogenic substances can be formed after you eat smoked, cured, or pickled foods that contain nitrites; they are also found in tobacco products.

Vitamin C is required for proper functioning of white blood cells in fighting infections, but smoking decreases the vitamin C levels inside these cells. The vitamin C levels of the white cells are also frequently diminished during infections and during periods of environmental, physical, or psychological stress.

Smoking one cigarette breaks down roughly the same amount of vitamin C as you would get from an orange. As a result, smokers have 30 to 50 percent less vitamin C in their bloodstreams than nonsmokers.

Fresh fruits and vegetables—especially citrus fruits, green peppers, cantaloupe, and broccoli—are the best sources of vitamin C. A number of studies suggest that the diets of many Americans, smokers and nonsmokers alike, contain suboptimal levels of this vitamin. Smokers take in less vitamin C than nonsmokers, even though they have a greater need for it. Smokers who do not eat breakfast are even more likely to be deficient in vitamin C. Thus, health-concerned smokers who do not already eat plenty of foods rich in vitamin C may be well advised either to add more vitamin C to their diets or to consider taking vitamin C supplements.

There is no evidence of a meaningful difference between "natural" and "synthetic" forms of this vitamin. One of the most convenient and least expensive ways to take vitamin C is in granular, rather than tablet, form. Granular vitamin C is a grainy powder usually taken dissolved in water or juice.

Vitamin C should be used with caution by persons with gout or kidney disease, since it may cause uric acid stones in the former and calcium oxalate stones in the latter. If you are planning to undergo screening for colon cancer, stop taking vitamin C for at least three days, since it can interfere with the accuracy of this test.[22]

Vitamin E

Vitamin E is an antioxidant that can protect laboratory animals against some toxic substances. Vitamin E can help block the formation of nitrosamines from substances found in tobacco smoke. It also seems to protect lung tissue and the vitamin A in your body from the effects of other oxidants in tobacco smoke. Vitamin E deficient rats are more sensitive to damage by cigarette smoke.

Large amounts of vitamin E can help protect laboratory animals from polluted air, probably because it protects the unsaturated fatty acids in the lung tissue from oxidation. It also increases the tumor-inhibiting ability of the mineral selenium (see below). Vitamin E may also help inhibit a precancerous breast condition in humans.

Vitamin E is a free radical scavenger. It neutralizes free radicals, which could cause damage to other cells and tissues if vitamin E did not "soak them up." Vitamin E may also protect against free radical damage to the cardiac muscles.

Vitamin E is generally considered safe in doses under 600 IUs. Possible overdose side effects include nausea, gas, diarrhea, fatigue, skin disorders, and slow healing of cuts or burns. Persons with high blood pressure, those taking anticoagulant drugs, and those with bleeding or clotting disorders should consult with their physician before taking vitamin E supplements. These supplements should be taken as part of a balanced vitamin/mineral preparation that includes selenium. Vitamin E should *not* be taken at the same time as birth control pills or inorganic iron supplements, as both can interfere with vitamin E activity.[23]

Selenium

Very small quantities of the trace material selenium are essential to human health. Selenium is required for the synthesis of the protective enzyme glutathione peroxidase, which protects cell membranes against damage by oxidants, including those in cigarette smoke. Selenium also seems to make platelets less sticky, decreasing the risk of heart attacks and strokes. It may also boost cellular immunity.

There is now a large body of evidence to suggest a connection between countries with selenium-rich soils and low cancer rates. Studies show that healthy people have higher selenium blood levels than cancer patients. It thus appears that selenium supplements, either in the diet or added to the drinking water, offer protection against a variety of forms of cancer.

Studies on the protective effects of selenium have generated a great deal of excitement among researchers. It has been the most widely studied mineral in recent years. High selenium levels in the diet have been found to inhibit the induction of a variety of cancers (skin, liver, colon, breast) in laboratory animals, while low selenium levels may be an additional cancer risk factor. Selenium also helps detoxify some of the heavy metals in cigarette smoke, such as mercury and cadmium.

A study led by Dr. Walter Willett of the Harvard School of Public Health found that people who came down with certain types of cancer had low selenium blood levels several years prior to the discovery of their cancers.

Dr. Gerald Schrauzer, a longtime selenium researcher at the University of California, San Diego, believes that the evidence that selenium can help protect against cancer is strong enough to suggest that virtually everyone should be sure they are receiving adequate amounts of this mineral.

The best dietary sources of selenium include organ meats (extremely high in selenium), seafood, beef, pork, lamb, and chicken (very high in selenium), broccoli, cabbage, celery, cucumbers, onions, mushrooms, radishes, brewer's yeast and grains. However, the selenium content of vegetables may vary over 100-fold depending on the region in which they were grown.

Selenium supplements are available in both inorganic and organic forms. Some researchers believe that the organic forms have fewer toxic effects. In addition, the absorption of inorganic selenium, particularly sodium selenite, may be decreased in the presence of vitamin C. The National Cancer Institute currently recommends a dietary intake of 50 to 200 micrograms of selenium per day as a cancer prevention measure.

Selenium can be toxic if doses larger than 200 micrograms per day are taken regularly. Symptoms of selenium toxicity include fragile or darkened fingernails, a metallic taste in the mouth, a metallic or garlicky breath, nausea, and dizziness.

Thus, especially for smokers, making sure you get enough selenium would seem a prudent pro-health measure. But even though the evidence that selenium may help prevent cancer is very encouraging, smokers should *not* think of selenium supplements as a magic anticancer pill. At best, it is extremely unlikely that selenium could completely reverse the harmful effects of tobacco smoke.[24]

Vitamin B_{12}

This vitamin helps to detoxify the cyanide found in tobacco smoke. Smokers excrete more B_{12} and thus have lower serum levels. This smoking-produced B_{12} deficiency is thought to be responsible for a disease called tobacco amblyopia. Tobacco amblyopia can produce dimming of vision in the central part of one's visual field. In some cases complete vision loss can occur. Tobacco amblyopia is treated with large doses of vitamin B_{12}. In addition to visual loss, patients with tobacco amblyopia may have difficulty distinguishing between red and green. The disease is most common in males who are heavy pipe smokers.

The recommended intake of vitamin B_{12} is 5 to 50 micrograms.[25]

Indoles and Isothiocyanates

These are cancer inhibitors found in high concentrations in the cruciferous vegetables (broccoli, cauliflower, cabbage, and brussels sprouts). Researchers believe that these substances may be necessary components of enzymes that detoxify carcinogens.[26]

Calcium

There is some evidence to suggest that taking in adequate levels of calcium may help decrease one's risk of colon cancer.[27]

Fiber

Dietary fiber is made of indigestible food fibers that create bulk in the bowels. In populations that consume large quantities of high-fiber foods, cancer of the colon is rare. Rates of colon cancer have increased over the years as the American diet has moved away from high-fiber whole foods and toward low-fiber processed foods. Among western countries in which large quantities of such refined foods as white bread, white flour, and white rice are eaten, colon cancer rates are quite high. Fiber is also a good preventive and treatment for constipation.

Many researchers recommend that westerners should try to double the fiber in their diet by adding such high-fiber foods as wheat bran, oat bran, bran cereals, and shredded wheat.

One of the reasons it's a good idea to get as many nutrients as possible from whole foods rather than vitamin supplements is that many high nutrient foods—whole grains, broccoli, peas, apples, beans, spinach, corn, etc.—also supply fiber. It's also possible to add fiber-rich food supplements as wheat brain, oat bran, and bran cereals to other foods.[28]

Should Smokers Take Vitamin and Mineral Supplements?

The question of whether to take vitamin supplements is a sticky one indeed. Some conservative researchers downplay the need for vitamin supplements and insist that a "balanced diet" can provide all our nutritional needs. While this is theoretically true, and while it *is* better to get our vitamins and minerals from the foods we eat, the fact is that many Americans do *not* receive the recommended levels of many vitamins and minerals from their diets. Few of us eat balanced diets, and many of our nutrients are grown on mineral-depleted soils. On the other hand, vitamin salesmen frequently make grandiose but unsubstantiated claims for their products.

One of the most even-handed commentators on this controversy is Sheldon Saul Hendler, M.D., Ph.D., an instructor at the University of California School of Medicine, San Diego. Dr. Hendler, who is both a biochemical researcher and a practicing physician, recently reviewed the medical literature, assessing the claims of both vitamin proponents and vitamin critics. His book, *The Complete Guide to Anti-Aging Nutrients*, is an island of reason in the midst of a confusing controversy. On the question of whether smokers should take vitamins, Dr. Hendler concludes:

"Smokers and nonsmokers regularly exposed to cigarette smoke could certainly benefit from increased antioxidant protection. Such protection is afforded by substances such as vitamin A (preferably beta-carotene), vitamin E, ascorbic acid (vitamin C), zinc, copper, selenium, and magnesium." Dr. Hendler recommends that smokers and nonsmokers alike could benefit from a two-pronged nutritional attack: Eat the best possible diet you can *and* take a daily "vitamin and mineral insurance" type of supplement.

Dr. Hendler's specific recommendations for smokers are as follows:[29]

Vitamins	Recommended Form	Amount	% RDA
Vitamin A*	beta-carotene	20,000 IU	400
Vitamin B_1	thiamine	10 mg	667
Vitamin B_2	riboflavin	10 mg	588
Niacinamide	niacinamide	100 mg	500
Pantothenic Acid	calcium pantothenate	50 mg	500
Vitamin B_{12}	cyanocobalamin	6 mcg	100
Biotin	biotin	100 mcg	33
Folic Acid	folic acid	400 mcg	100
Vitamin C	ascorbic acid	1,000 mg	1,666
Vitamin E	d-alpha tocopheryl acetate	400 IU	1,330
Vitamin D_3	cholecalciferol	400 IU	100

Minerals	Recommended Form	Amount	% RDA
Calcium †	carbonate	1,000 mg	125
Copper	gluconate	3 mg	150
Chromium	organic form/chromium yeast	100 mcg	‡
Magnesium	gluconate preferred/oxide acceptable	400 mg	100
Manganese	gluconate	5 mg	‡
Molybdenum	sodium molybdate	50 mg	‡
Selenium	organic form/selenium yeast	200 mg	‡
Zinc	gluconate	30 mg	200
Iodine	potassium iodide	150 mcg	100
Women add:			
Iron	sulfate or fumarate	18 mg	100

*If you are taking preformed vitamin A rather than beta-carotene, do not take more than 15,000 IU. Pregnant women should take no more than 5,000 IU of preformed vitamin A.

†1,500 mg of calcium per day is recommended for postmenopausal women. Only 40 percent of calcium carbonate is free calcium, so a calcium carbonate dose of 2,500 mg. would be required to produce a free calcium dose of 1,000 mg.

‡U.S. RDA not determined.

Where can you find such a vitamin and mineral insurance formula? Dr. Hendler recommends the following. (Current prices and formulas are available from both companies on request. Neither Dr. Hendler nor anyone involved in writing or publishing *The No-Nag, No-Guilt, Do-It-Your-Own-Way Guide to Quitting Smoking* has any economic interest in these companies.)

NutriGuard Research
238 Lolita Street
Encinitas, CA 92024.
Recommended product: Broad Spectrum Formula

Bronson Pharmaceuticals
4526 Rinetti Lane
La Canada, CA 91011
Recommended products:
    Vitamin and Mineral Insurance Formula;
    Fortified Vitamin and Mineral Insurance Formula

In addition, smokers who are members of the following groups may have other special needs for vitamins and minerals:

- Women using oral contraceptives.
- Pregnant women.
- Postmenopausal women.
- People on weight-loss diets.
- Runners and other athletes.
- People who drink significant quantities of alcoholic beverages.
- Hospitalized patients.
- People exposed to high levels of environmental pollutants.
- Older people.

Dr. Hendler's book, *The Complete Guide to Anti-Aging Nutrients*, provides additional guidelines for each of these groups.

Fat

In addition to *increasing* their intake of the nutrients listed above, health-concerned smokers would be wise to substantially *decrease* their intake of the one food most hazardous to health—fat.

The National Academy of Sciences committee that in 1982 reviewed the scientific literature of the link between diet and cancer, concluded that of all the nutrients in Americans' diet, the one most strongly linked to cancer was fat. It was well known that reducing dietary fat can help you reduce your risk of heart disease, but recent studies suggest that cutting down on fat can cut your cancer risk as well. Dietary fat is a major contributor to breast, colon, and rectal cancers. One study estimated that 27 percent of breast cancers are caused by high-fat diets. Polyunsaturated fats, while better for heart disease, may be worse for cancer. It is now believed that monounsaturated fats—such as olive oil—may also prevent heart disease. The wisest approach now seems to be to significantly reduce the amount of animal fat in your diet (of the type found in meat, butter, and cheese) while continuing to eat moderate levels of monounsaturated (olive oil) and unsaturated (corn and safflower oil) fats from vegetable sources.[30]

All-Star Foods:

These foods have high levels of one or more of the nutrients recommended in this chapter:

broccoli	cauliflower
cabbage	brussels sprouts
cantaloupe	carrots
bran	whole grains
fruits	sweet potatoes

Eating Quiz for Health-Concerned Smokers

1. How many times per week do you eat red meat?
   (a) none   (b) 1–3   (c) 4–6   (d) 7–10
   (e) more than 10

2. How many times per week do you eat preserved or processed meats (hot dogs, bologna, bacon, luncheon meats, etc.)?
   (a) none   (b) 1–2   (c) 3–4   (d) 5–6
   (e) more than 6

3. How many times per week do you eat fried or deep-fried foods?
   (a) none   (b) 1–2   (c) 3–4   (d) 5–6
   (e) more than 6

4. How many times per week do you eat cheese? (Do not count low-fat cottage cheese.)
   (a) none   (b) 1–2   (c) 3–4   (d) 5–6
   (e) more than 6

5. How many servings of vegetables do you eat per day?
   (a) 4 or more   (b) 3   (c) 2   (d) 1
   (e) none

6. How many servings of the cruciferous vegetables do you eat per week (broccoli, cauliflower, brussels sprouts, cabbage, greens, turnips, rutabagas)?
   (a) 7 or more   (b) 5–6   (c) 3–4   (d) 1–2
   (e) none

7. How many servings of fresh fruit or fruit juice do you have per day?
   (a) 4 or more   (b) 3   (c) 2   (d) 1
   (e) none

8. How many servings of fruits and vegetables high in vitamin A do you normally eat per week (apricots, cantaloupe, broccoli, carrots, greens, pumpkin, spinach, sweet potatoes, winter squash)?
   (a) 7 or more   (b) 5–6   (c) 3–4   (d) 1–2
   (e) none

9. What kind of milk do you drink?
   (a) skim or none (b) ½–1%   (c) 1–1½%   (d) 2%
   (e) whole

10. How many pats of butter do you use per day?
    (a) none   (b) ½   (c) 1   (d) 2–3
    (e) 4 or more

SCORING: Give yourself 5 points for each (a) answer, 4 for (b),
3 for (c), 2 for (d), and 1 for (e).

46–50   You're doing terrific. Keep it up. Congratulations!
41–45   You're doing great. Keep up the good work and
           consider some minor improvements.
31–40   You're doing pretty well, but there's still some
           room for improvement.
21–30   You're making an effort, but could benefit greatly
           from additional improvements.
10–20   You could substantially improve your health and
           reduce your health risks by making some dietary
           changes.

III. STRESS CONTROL

Have you ever wondered why some people seem to thrive
on challenge, responsibility, and adversity while others
have difficulty managing the stresses of ordinary life?
Kenneth R. Pelletier, Ph.D., author of the stress classic
Mind as Healer, Mind as Slayer, believes that the key to
managing stress effectively is to alternate intense periods
of purposeful activity with periods of "time off" from
all tasks, responsibilities, and worries. "Successful stress
managers have learned to provide themselves with periodic *islands of peace*—little daily 'stress vacations' that
help them break the cycle of chronic stress," says Dr.
Pelletier, who is an associate clinical professor at the
University of California School of Medicine, San Francisco.

"For many smokers, having a cigarette provides just
such an island of peace," he continues. "When they light
up, all their other worries, all the petty hassles of life, are
temporarily set aside. It is this factor—in combination with

the pharmacological actions of nicotine—that makes smoking such a valuable tool in dealing with stress. Smokers who wish to cut down or quit simply need to establish *other* islands of peace in their lives," Pelletier advises. "After all, nonsmokers have found a thousand ways to break the stress cycle without having a cigarette. Health-concerned smokers can learn to do likewise."

Pelletier suggests that health-concerned smokers can go through a 7-step do-it-yourself process of stress reduction:

1. Understand the key stressors in your life.
2. Identify your particular stress signals.
3. Create islands of peace in your everyday schedule.
4. Explore new relaxation possibilities and choose the best.
5. Rehearse and visualize your relaxation plan.
6. Put your plan into action.
7. Modify and adapt your plan as needed.

Understanding Your Key Stressors

When you find yourself under stress, Pelletier suggests a three-step approach: "Number one: *Don't panic.* Number two: Consciously sit down and plan a number of quiet, peaceful activities over the next hours, days, and weeks. Number three: Look for ways to use your whole range of stress resources—exercise, quiet time, social support, massage, a healthy diet, inspiration, enjoyment, laughter, a strong sense of purpose, a rich spiritual life, and so on, *to nickle-and-dime your stress hazards to death.*"

It's useful to think in terms of two kinds of stress: short-term and long-term. A short-term stress reaction is the appropriate and healthy response to an emergency situation.

Here's an example from my own life: Several years ago I was working on my car and needed to leave the transmission in neutral with the brake off. I was parked on a hill, so I put bricks under the two front tires. When I finished my work, I neglected to put the brake back on.

Several hours later I came out of the house, kicked the bricks out from under the tires, then watched in horror as my brand-new car began to roll slowly down the hill. I grabbed at the passenger-side door, but it was locked. The car continued to gather speed. There was a steep drop-off at the bottom of the hill.

Somehow—exactly how I'll never know—I managed to run all the way around the accelerating car, open the driver's door, jump in, and step on the brake. The car skidded to a stop a few feet from the precipice. I never knew I could move so quickly. I sat there in the driver's seat for a good fifteen minutes afterward, totally spent, my arms and legs shaking.

If I'd been hooked up to a stress level monitor when my car began rolling down the hill, it would have shown a curve that looked like this:

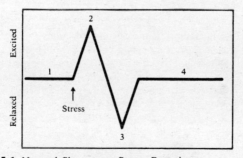

Figure 5-1 Normal Short-term Stress Reaction
Point 1 is a baseline stress level before the emergency situation. Point 2 is a normal stress reaction. Point 3 corresponds to the post-stress period of compensatory relaxation. Point 4 indicates a return to baseline stress.

"With a short-term stress response you encounter the
stressor, you deal with it, then there's a period of relaxation, giving you a chance to recover," Pelletier explains. "In a short-term stress reaction, the source of
stress is immediate, identifiable, and resolvable. The
stressor may be an argument with your spouse, an over-
due bill, a disappointment at work, or a tight deadline.
Most of us experience many stressful events per day. In
most cases we can take appropriate steps to deal with the
stressor, then give ourselves a chance to relax and recover."

Thus, over a longer period of time, our stress level
might look like this:

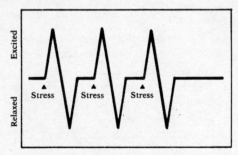

Figure 5-2 Repeated Short-term Stress Reactions
This pattern reflects a period in which a person was
able to deal with a series of stressful events using a
short-term reaction. After dealing with each stressor,
the subject allowed herself a period of compensatory
relaxation. Thus by the time the next stressor oc-
curred, she had returned to her baseline stress level.

But sometimes we do not handle stress so well. We
may find ourself in a situation in which it seems that the
stressors come so quickly that we do not have a chance
to recover from the last one before the next one occurs.

The worst kind of stresses are those that are *not* easily
identifiable and *not* easily resolvable in the short term.

But the "islands of peace" principle can help us deal more effectively even with these more severe life stresses—a major upset in our work life, the loss of an important relationship, a chronic illness, or continuing financial difficulties.

We get into trouble when our short-term stress cycle does not get a chance to complete itself and stressful events begin to pile up. This pushes us into the realm of long-term stress. When we are in a state of long-term stress, the next stressful event occurs before we have fully recovered from the last one. A typical long-term stress pattern might look like this:

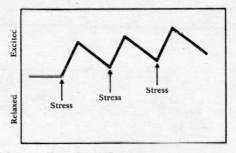

Figure 5-3 Long-Term Stress Pattern
There are three things wrong with maintaining a long-term stress pattern: It's not much fun; it makes us less productive; it puts us at increased risk of accidents, illness, or injury.

It is when they find themselves in such long-term stress patterns that smokers rely most heavily on their cigarettes. But smoking provides only temporary relief. It can help smokers repress—rather than deal with—feelings of anger and sadness. It can help them ignore—rather than take steps to deal with—an unsatisfactory work or home environment.

One smoker we interviewed compared smoking in the midst of a crisis to using a Band-Aid to treat a broken bone: It gives you the illusion that you are in control of the situation while encouraging you to ignore the root of the problem.

If long-term stress patterns continue, they can lead to an illness, accident, or psychological breakdown that forces the individual into a period of quiet recuperation. According to an estimate by the National Institute of Occupational Safety and Health, 60 to 80 percent of industrial accidents are stress-related.[31]

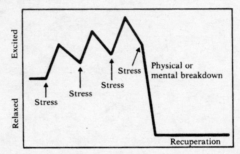

Figure 5-4 Long-Term Stress Pattern Leading to Breakdown
The longer a long-term stress pattern continues, the greater the chance that it will be resolved by a physical or psychological breakdown.

Identifying Your Stress Signals

"We all have our own unique stress signals," Pelletier explains. "The first two things I usually notice are a tightness in the muscles of my upper back and an increasing impatience."

Here are some other common stress signals:

- digestive upset
- headaches
- insomnia
- loss of appetite
- feelings of hopelessness

- eating binges
- increased distractibility
- increased alcohol or drug use
- grouchiness and irritability
- increased smoking

Take a minute to identify your own stress signals: Think back to the last time you found yourself feeling extremely stressed. Close your eyes and remember how you felt and how your stress manifested itself during that period.

Creating Your Own Nonsmoking "Islands Of Peace"

Modern society generates many chronic stresses. But there's usually a way to break the frantic cycle and establish islands of peace and tranquility in our lives. Many of us have already developed very effective ways of finding some relaxation and peace. Some like to listen to music. Some engage in sports. Others pursue a craft or hobby.

Overburdened parents can arrange to swap child-care time with other parents. People who must drive long distances to work may be able to shift their work time to avoid rush hour. Those who are chronically disorganized can invest in a good book on time management—I suggest Alan Lakein's *How to Get Control of Your Time and Your Life*[32]—and use a time planning notebook[33] to help them organize their days.

Other tips for scheduling your own "islands of peace":

- Schedule blocks of quiet time well in advance. Write them down in your appointment book.

- Look at your schedule for the upcoming week.

Block out at least one evening to be reserved for an enjoyable, nonwork related activity, something you will really look forward to.

- Schedule time for phone calls to people you care about.

- Set up lunch dates with friends. Ideally these should be people who have nothing to do with your work, people with whom you can talk about personal matters.

- Look for opportunities to take short breaks: A quick walk. Five minutes of stretching exercises. A quiet cup of tea.

- Be on the lookout for opportunities to become physically quiet: A brief nap. A bath or shower. Getting a back rub or massage.

- Exercise can be a great stress breaker. When you're feeling tense, there's nothing better than a long, slow jog, a long hike in the park, or a stint of gardening or yard work.

- Interacting with pets can be a wonderful way to relax. Taking your dog for a walk combines both companionship and exercise. There are few things more satisfying than sitting quietly with a purring cat in your lap.

- You are the best judge of relaxation methods. Take a blank piece of paper and give yourself five minutes to brainstorm possible ways to establish islands of peace in *your* life.

Exploring New Options

When deadlines and demands pile up, many of us tend to skip rather than increase the activities that allow our bodies to restore themselves. Once you've begun to establish some islands of peace in your daily routine, they will help serve as beachheads against the "full-court press" of life. They will give you a time and space to realize that you don't really *need* to depend on cigarettes to relax.

Making long-term changes requires time. Don't be in a hurry. Simply begin to cultivate the little spaces and gaps in your day-to-day life—and to fill them with non-smoking activities. Is this a good time for a walk? A stretch break? Would an afternoon nap work for you? Here are some solutions that have proved useful to others:

A social worker: "I see clients for most of my working day, and the phone was always ringing. I realized I was getting most of my calls between nine and ten in the morning and four and five in the afternoon, so I started keeping that time free for the phone and turned on the answering machine from ten to four. It worked like a charm."

A salesman: "The biggest hassle of my day was being stuck in traffic. I shifted my hours around to miss the worst of it, and rented some tape-recorded books to listen to when I'm driving. Now I'm actually sometimes sorry when I get where I'm going."

A housewife: "I realized that I really *did* drink too much coffee. It gave me a quick burst of energy, but I paid for it later. I stocked my home with mineral water and switched to decaf except for one cup at breakfast and one after lunch. This works much better for me."

A nurse: "I realized I was getting home from work tense, going directly to the refrigerator and just pigging out. I started taking a hot bath first and planning my menus in advance. I feel a lot better and I've already lost five pounds."

A journalist: "When I'm on a deadline, I get really stressed out and stop running. I tell myself, gee, I'm so darn busy, I don't have time to run today. Then, of course, I'd feel all that much worse because I hadn't gotten any exercise. I started exercising on my way home from work, no matter what, even if it was just a quiet twenty-minute walk in the park.''

Rehearsing Your New Patterns

If you watched the last Olympics, you probably saw some of the world's top athletes sitting quietly with eyes closed just before their event began. They were visualizing every step of their performance. You can use the same technique. Pick the most important stress reduction ideas that occur to you in your observation period and begin to think about exactly how you would put them into practice.

Use your islands of peace to rehearse these new activities. Think your proposed activities through, step by step—see yourself driving to work earlier to miss the crowds. It's darker and colder and there's a lot less traffic. Or visualize yourself spending your Saturday at home puttering around the house and working in the garden instead of going to work.

Once you have visualized your new relaxing activity, take the final step and let yourself actually *do* it. For as long as it takes, put all your energy into getting the ball rolling. Do everything you can to ensure your success—this will help you build up a good head of steam, so that you can go on to make other positive changes later.

Self-Understanding

"The most effective steps in reducing our stress levels don't require a lot of technical expertise," Pelletier says. "But they *do* require a good measure of self-understanding. It is difficult for many of us to understand why, even though we *know* many things we *could* do to reduce our stress level, we don't *do* them. I believe that on some deep level it's because we feel we don't *deserve* it.

"The truth is, we *do* deserve it. In the end the key to do-it-yourself stress relief is accepting the fact that it's O.K. for us to nurture ourselves. It's O.K.—even necessary—for us to care for ourselves. By accepting this right—and this responsibility—we'll be taking a giant step toward a calmer, more centered life."[34]

IV. SOCIAL SUPPORT

In addition to its other characteristics, smoking is a form of communication. It's no accident that in the movie *White Nights*, Mikhail Baryshnikov makes smoking a cigarette an essential part of a dance performance. Smoking *is* a kind of dance. Taking the cigarette out of the pack, handling it, lighting it, drawing in the smoke, feeling it in your throat and lungs, blowing it out, watching the smoke disperse—each part of the process becomes an intricate and meaningful communicative gesture. When two people smoke together, it can serve as a kind of ceremony, a shared experience. This is not something to be given up lightly.

Social support plays an extremely important role in smoking behavior. Smokers who receive social support to cut down or quit will have an easier time modifying their smoking behavior. Health-concerned smokers may find it particularly difficult to control their smoking habits *unless they are able to arrange social support for the changes they wish to make*. As one successful quitter told us: "I can practically guarantee that smokers who ignore the social dimension of smoking will have little luck in taking control of their habit." Many researchers feel that social support is *the* key to taking control of your smoking.

Social support is an extremely important factor in *any* effort to change one's behavior. Studies of inactive people who decided to begin exercising found that those with the greatest social support were most successful. The kind of social support that seems to be most effective is that of your spouse, close family members, and closest friends. One research team found that their subjects' patterns of adherence to an exercise regimen was directly related to the spouses' attitudes toward the program.[35]

In smoking, social support plays a key role from the very beginning. Most smokers take up the habit in their teen years. During this time, teenagers are working hard to distance themselves from the influence of their parents. They are establishing stronger links with their peers, and are striving to assert their independence.

Smoking is attractive to them because it allows them to feel independent and grown-up and serves as a bond with their smoking friends. Studies show that nearly 90 percent of teenage smokers have one or more close friends who smoke—compared to only 33 percent of nonsmoking teens. The child of two smoking parents is twice as likely to smoke as the child of two nonsmokers.[36]

Smokers who wish to cut down or quit can benefit greatly by getting support from the key people in their lives. It is also a good idea to identify friends or family members who may be *disturbed* by your efforts to modify your smoking behavior and who may therefore try to impede your progress.

Take a minute now to list the names of the most important people in your life—your spouse, your closest family members, friends, and other key people. Give each one a score on a scale of 1 to 10, with 10 indicating that this person is completely supportive of your efforts to control your smoking, and 1 indicating that he or she is totally resistant. Here's one smoker's list:

Sheldon P.'s Key Support People

Marilyn	9
Mother	10
Uncle Jay	2
Aunt Julia	8
Carlos	10
Minnie	4
Allen	8
Howard	3
Carla	1

It will be important for you to forge strong bonds with the people who are most supportive of your efforts to control your smoking. You may also wish to take steps to make yourself less vulnerable to the pressures from those who may be threatened or disturbed by your desire to make this change.

Dealing with Nonsupportive Friends

It is probably wise to say little or nothing about your plans to the friends you think would be bothered by your decision to cut down or quit. In the example cited above, Sheldon's Uncle Jay and his friend Carla are both heavy smokers who show little interest in changing their smok-

ing patterns. Thus, it is unlikely that either of them will
be an effective support person in the smoker's efforts to
do so. On the other hand, Sheldon's wife, his mother,
and a coworker have all encouraged him to take steps to
reduce his health risks and have indicated their willingness to help in any way they can.

Don't be surprised if you find that some of your friends,
especially those who are smokers themselves, end up trying to sabotage your efforts to cut down or quit. Things
may be especially difficult if your spouse or other close
friends and family members are disturbed by the changes
you intend to make. Your success in these efforts might
make them more uncomfortable with their own smoking.
Or they may feel that your efforts to control your smoking
will put a strain on your friendship. As one team of
smoking researchers has written, "It is not uncommon
to see a husband who is ostensibly encouraging his wife
to cut down, approaching her, cigarette pack extended,
saying, 'Here, it's been a long time since you've had
one.' Business associates, too, may razz you about quitting and try to foist cigarettes on you."[37]

Try to understand such apparently hostile behavior as
best you can. If your friends *do* razz you or offer you
cigarettes, try not to get angry. Just be as understanding
and patient as you can. You may wish to say something
like: "Bob, I'm trying to cut down. I'd appreciate it if
you wouldn't offer me cigarettes."

In some cases it may be necessary to temporarily avoid
a few of your nonsupportive smoking friends until you
have reached the smoking control goal you have set for
yourself. Two of the most common reasons for failure in
smoking control efforts are socializing with smoking
friends and the use of alcohol.

How Friends Can Help

Fortunately, most smokers have a number of close friends and family members who would be only too happy to help them cut down or quit. It's a good idea to begin talking with these potential supporters as early as possible about your plans to take control of your smoking. If you are lucky enough to have friends who have quit smoking, you may find them a particularly good source of support. They've been through it, they know how it feels, and they can offer useful tips and moral support.

Ask your most supportive friends if they would be willing to help. If they agree, be specific about what they can do. For instance, you might ask them to:

- Provide a reward for meeting one or more of your smoking control goals.

- Take you out to lunch or dinner once a week while you're putting your smoking control program into action.

- Call or visit regularly to see how you're doing.

- Be available by phone 24 hours a day during the toughest parts of your smoking control program.

Avoiding Smoking Situations

Studies show that being in the presence of other smokers is a powerful inducement to smoke.[38] Smokers who are trying to control their habit should do their best to avoid all situations in which others are smoking. This may require some changes in your present habits. For example:

- Ask to be seated in the nonsmoking section of restaurants.

- Ask others not to smoke in your presence.

- Post a small NO SMOKING sign by your front door. Provide an outside area where smokers may go if they wish to smoke.

- If you are in a group and others light up, excuse yourself, and don't return until they have finished.

- Do not buy, carry, light, or hold cigarettes for others.

Cutting Down with a Buddy

There is much to be said for cutting down or quitting with a spouse, a friend, or a group of friends. Two or more health-concerned smokers can provide important mutual assistance for each other. Your buddy will be a sympathetic and understanding listener when you are going through the difficult times of changing your smoking patterns. And a bit of healthy competition doesn't hurt. No one wants to be the one who fails while a buddy succeeds.

Pomerleau and Pomerleau suggest that "Ground Rule number one in any smoking group should be: 'Ignore failure, praise success.' " Your buddies should not feel that they can arouse more attention or interest for lapses than for positive achievements.[39]

Until recently, the pervading culture in most western countries was very supportive of smoking: Smoking was considered the norm. Ashtrays were always provided. A cigarette was considered a sign of sophistication.

Although smoking is still the norm in some social groups, many Americans, especially urban, well-educated professionals, have declared their homes and

cars no-smoking areas. Smokers who move in these circles are now much more likely to feel that they are of-
fending nonsmokers by their habit. And smoking is now
receiving considerably less favorable treatment in virtually all contemporary media.

As one team of smoking researchers writes, "As the
issue of smoking becomes more important in daily life
and as more antismoking messages become obvious, the
likelihood increases that individuals will want to quit
smoking and that they will succeed."[40]

Using Professional Support

As part of your effort to take more control of your smoking, you may wish to schedule one or more sessions with
your physician, your minister or other spiritual advisor,
or with a therapist or counselor.

If you *do* decide to visit your physician, do ask your
doctor to give you a stern picture of the negative effects
of smoking on your health, including an estimate of how
many years of healthy life you might forfeit by continuing to smoke. Studies show that receiving forceful advice
from a physician helps increase your chances of success.

Some communities have established telephone support
services for health-concerned smokers: A new antismoking message is recorded each day. Health-concerned
smokers can call the hotline number whenever they wish
and listen to the message.[41] You can call the American
Lung Association's Rochester Freedom Line to listen to
their current message at 1-716-442-3219.

Using a Support Group

You may wish to find out what smoking control groups there are in your area. Look under Smokers' Information and Treatment Centers in your local Yellow Pages. In addition, be sure to check listings under Health Agencies, Health Clubs, and Physical Fitness. National organizations that sponsor local programs include the American Cancer Society and the American Lung Association. In addition, many Seventh Day Adventist pastors have had special training in facilitating smoking control groups. In many communities, the local Seventh Day Adventist Church will supply a leader for a group of smokers you put together yourself. (Their programs are nondenominational, with an optional spiritual component.) Addresses for these groups are listed in chapter 10.

Cutting Down for Someone Else

When we started our research for *The No-Nag, No-Guilt, Do-It-Your-Own-Way Guide to Quitting Smoking*, I placed a classified ad in the magazine I edit, *Medical Self-Care*, asking our readers to send in tips or advice for health-concerned smokers. One of the most memorable responses was from a woman in California, who wrote:

> Twenty-seven years ago, when my sister was born, both my parents smoked three packs of unfiltered Camel cigarettes per day. By the time she was three weeks old, my sister had suffered five major asthma attacks. The doctor told my parents that their cigarette smoke was aggravating her condition. As soon as they left the doctor's office, they agreed to quit smoking.

My mother told me that she walked a hundred miles during those first few weeks. She learned all the cracks in the sidewalk. My father bought gum by the carton and chewed it until his jaws ached. It was hard, but they persevered. And they made it. Neither of them ever smoked again.

The thought I'd like to offer your health-concerned smokers is just this: Perhaps if people don't love *themselves* enough to cut down on their smoking, they may love someone else enough to do it.

6
Controlled Smoking: Cutting Your Risk by Smoking Less

Health-concerned smokers may feel they have only two choices: quitting or continuing to smoke at their present level. But there *is* a third alternative—*controlled smoking.*

There are many smokers who, while they may feel either unwilling or unable to quit right now, *are* willing—even eager—to take steps to reduce their health risks. Controlled smoking is simply a strategy for continuing to smoke in a way that minimizes the consumption of tobacco—and thus reduces the negative health effects associated with smoking. One of the greatest appeals of this approach is that it provides specific pro-health guidelines and techniques for health-concerned smokers who do not yet feel ready to quit.

Nicotine Compensation

Successfully controlling one's smoking is more than just a matter of decreasing the number of cigarettes smoked per day. When addicted smokers cut down, they unconsciously modify their puffing patterns in order to obtain more nicotine from each cigarette. In a recent study by San Francisco General Hospital researcher Neal Benowitz and his colleagues, smokers who cut down from an average of 37 cigarettes per day to an average of 5 cigarettes per day (with no special efforts to control their puffing patterns) increased their intake of smoke per cigarette by threefold. Thus although they cut their number of cigarettes by 86 percent, they decreased their overall smoke intake by only 50 percent. Thus smokers who wish to curtail their smoke intake must control both their *number of cigarettes smoked per day* and *the way they smoke each cigarette*. For more on nicotine compensation, see chapter 7.

Among smoking researchers, the concept of controlled smoking is considered quite controversial. Smoking researcher Russell Glasgow, one of the key developers of this method, puts it this way: "We see controlled smoking as an alternative for some smokers who wouldn't otherwise become engaged in attempts to change their smoking. I would still strongly emphasize that the best thing to do—and the ultimate goal— is to stop smoking altogether. But controlled smoking may be a useful step on the way to quitting for some smokers."

Steps to Controlled Smoking

The idea of controlled smoking was originally developed by psychologist Lee Fredericksen of the V.A. Medical Center in Jackson, Mississippi.[1] In recent years, the major figures in the field of controlled smoking have been Russell Glasgow of the Oregon Research Institute in Eugene, Oregon, Robert Klesges of Memphis State University, and their colleagues.[2] Glasgow and Klesges have developed a six-session program that gives smokers the option of either quitting entirely or learning the skills of controlled smoking. Their work demonstrates that many health-concerned smokers *can* substantially reduce their intake of cigarette smoke at least for a period of six to twelve months.[3]

The controlled smoking program emphasizes three principal strategies for decreasing the intake of tobacco smoke:

- Reducing the number of cigarettes smoked by one-half to two-thirds.
- Switching to a brand containing 50 percent or less of the nicotine of your present brand.
- Reducing the percentage of each cigarette smoked by one-half to two-thirds.

Smokers attend hour-long small group meetings led by a psychologist one evening a week for six weeks. The sections that follow provide guidelines for developing a similar program on your own.

WEEK ONE

Cut your nicotine intake by 50 percent by switching to a new brand of cigarettes. The steps listed below should make this easy:

1. Turn to Appendix IV, which shows the tar and nicotine content of all current U.S. cigarettes.
2. Find the nicotine content of the brand you presently smoke.
3. Choose two or three brands with approximately *half* the nicotine level of your current brand.
4. Buy a pack of *each* of the two or three brands you have chosen. Be sure to sample *each* of these lower-nicotine brands. This is important.
5. Choose one of these lower-nicotine brands as your new brand, and smoke only that new brand.

6. Buy a pocket notebook small enough to carry with you at all times. You may smoke whenever you wish, but be sure to record each cigarette you smoke—either before you light up or while you are smoking it. Do *not* wait until later to record your cigarettes.

Since you won't have a weekly meeting to go to if you're doing this on your own, Dr. Glasgow suggests that you ask a sympathetic friend to be your support person. Meet with this friend at least once a week to review your progress.

CASE STUDY: At the beginning of her program of controlled smoking, Cindy Daniels smoked Marlboro king-sized filter cigarettes, with a nicotine content of 1.0 mg per cigarette. After consulting Appendix IV, Cindy chose three brands with approximately half the nicotine content: Winston Ultra Lights (0.4 mg.), Tareyton Lights (0.4 mg), and Merit (0.5 mg). After buying and testing a pack of each of these three brands, Cindy chose Tareyton Lights as her new brand. She then recorded each cigarette she smoked in a pocket notebook.

Dr. Glasgow has found that although many smokers have tried to switch brands on their own, most are unsuccessful. The Glasgow-Klesges method works because (1) the smoker isn't making that large a change in nicotine level, (2) smokers are able to select a new brand from several alternative choices, and (3) smokers monitor the number of cigarettes smoked so that they don't unconsciously increase their number of cigarettes per day to compensate for the lower nicotine level.[4]

WEEKS TWO AND THREE

During your second and third weeks you will concentrate on reducing the number of cigarettes you smoke. To begin, look back over your notebook for the previous week and calculate the average number of cigarettes you smoked per day. Record that number in your pocket notebook. This is your former smoking level.

Now divide this number in half. This will give you your target smoking level. Record this number in your notebook.

> CASE STUDY: Cindy found that she had smoked an average of 28 cigarettes per day for the preceding week. Thus, her former and target smoking levels were as follows:
>
> *Former smoking level: 28 per day*
> *Target smoking level: 14 per day*

Dr. Glasgow emphasizes that cutting down on the number of cigarettes you smoke per day is the single most effective part of controlled smoking. Decreasing the number of cigarettes smoked decreases the harmful substances taken into the smoker's body. The number of cigarettes smoked per day is much easier to monitor than some of the other subtle parts of smoking behavior.

Dr. Glasgow and his colleagues offer the following strategies for cutting down to your target smoking level:

Make your cigarettes less accessible. Stop carrying your pack of cigarettes with you. Keep them in an unusual, distant place that requires thought, planning, and a special trip when you want to have one. Some people keep their cigarettes out in the garage. Others keep them in an out-of-the-way room. Another way to make your cigarettes less accessible is to have someone else—ideally a nonsmoking friend, family member, or coworker—keep your day's quota of cigarettes for you. Set it up so you *can* get a cigarette if you really want one, but make it a real hassle to do so.

One successful quitter told us that for the last few weeks before she quit altogether she kept her cigarettes in a sock at the bottom of the dirty laundry basket in the basement laundry room: "I had to *really* want a cigarette before I'd go down to that cold, clammy place to get one."

Give yourself a time limit. You may, for example, decide to limit yourself to no more than one cigarette per hour. Assuming that you sleep eight hours per night, this single step will reduce your number of cigarettes smoked to 16 per day.

Establish places or situations in which you will not smoke. You may wish to establish your car, your office, or your bedroom as a "non-smoking area." You may decide that you will not smoke while in the presence of nonsmokers, in friends' homes, while talking on the telephone, while driving, or while a passenger in another's car.

Use these—and other—strategies to reduce your daily number of cigarettes smoked until you reach your target smoking level of half your previous level. (Some smokers choose to cut down to one-third their former level.) Remember to continue to record each cigarette you smoke in your pocket notebook. Discuss your progress regularly with your support person.

WEEK FOUR

At this point, Dr. Glasgow's program offers smokers the option of quitting altogether. Some people find this easier than continuing the gradual reduction of smoking. And quitting should now be easier, since you have already switched brands and cut down substantially on your number of cigarettes smoked per day. If you wish to quit now, proceed to chapter 8.

If you prefer to continue your program of controlled smoking, you will spend this week becoming more aware of the length of your cigarette butts. Although this may seem somewhat obsessive, it does provide a simple way to reduce your intake of cigarette smoke.

Begin this week by collecting the butts of all the cigarettes you smoke in a day. Put them out carefully, so as not to "squash" them. You will now calculate the portion of each cigarette you actually smoke.

Using a ruler, measure the length of each butt, and take the average. This is your former butt length. Record this number in your pocket notebook.

Again using a ruler, measure an unsmoked cigarette. Record this number in your pocket notebook as the length of unsmoked cigarette. Subtract former butt length of unsmoked cigarette. The result is your former portion of cigarette smoked.

Now divide your former portion of cigarette smoked by 2. This will give you your target portion of cigarette to smoke.

CASE STUDY: Kevin's cigarettes were $3\frac{3}{8}$ inches long. His butts were $1\frac{3}{8}$ inches long. His notebook calculation looked like this:

Length of Unsmoked Cigarette 3⅜ inches	minus —	Former Butt Length 1⅜ inches	equals =	Former Portion of Cigarette Smoked 2 inches

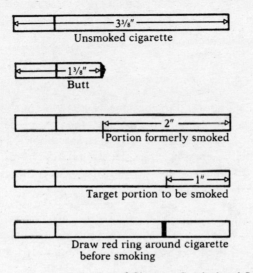

Figure 6-1 Calculating Portion of Cigarette Smoked and Setting a Reduced Target

Kevin's former portion of cigarette smoked was 2 inches. Thus, his target portion of cigarette to smoke was 1 inch.

Once you have obtained your own target portion of cigarette to smoke, take your ruler and a red marking pen and draw a circle around each of the remaining cigarettes in your pack, marking the place where you will stop smoking. For example, if your target portion is 1 inch, draw a circle around your cigarette 1 inch from the tip. From now on, each time you open a new pack, take all the cigarettes out and mark them in the same way.

This is very important. The red circles will help you make sure you don't forget and start smoking your cigarettes all the way down.

Note: Some nonfilter smokers may be tempted to simply cut their cigarettes in half. *Don't do this!* Shortened, unfiltered cigarettes produce higher levels of tar per puff than uncut ones.

WEEK FIVE

It is now important to consider whether you may be compensating for your low-nicotine brand, your decreased number of cigarettes, and your decreased portion of each cigarette by inhaling more deeply, taking more frequent puffs, by compressing the filter, or by covering the ventilating holes or grooves.

At this point, please take a few minutes to read or review the section on nicotine compensation in chapter 7. Once you have done so, take this opportunity to look back over the four previous weeks of controlled smoking and review the progress you have made up to this point. Here are the methods you have used to date:

- Switching to a lower-nicotine brand.
- Reducing the number of cigarettes smoked.
- Reducing the portion of each cigarette smoked.

Now select *one* on these three components to work on further during the fifth week. Most of the subjects in Dr. Glasgow's study chose to continue to further decrease the number of cigarettes smoked per day.

WEEK SIX

Review your progress to date. What was your biggest success? Your biggest disappointment? Be aware that a very common occurrence is something researchers call the goal violation effect. This is the tendency, upon failing to fulfill one's goal 100 percent on the first try, to become discouraged, abandon one's efforts, and return to one's former smoking level. This effect is frequently observed in people who want to lose weight: They put themselves on an unrealistically rigorous diet, and after the first lapse, give up completely and proceed to eat their former amounts or even more than ever.

Remember, one failure does not mean you will never succeed. The best baseball players in the world get on base *less than half the time!* Don't let occasional setbacks keep you from persevering in your efforts to reduce your smoking risks.

Take a few moments to review your progress and to think about where you wish to go from here. You have three alternatives:

- You may decide to continue to reduce your daily intake of tobacco smoke by the methods described above.
- You may decide to continue to smoke at your present reduced level.
- You may decide to quit smoking altogether.

Here are the actual choices made by the members of Dr. Glasgow's and Dr. Klesges's workshop:

Continued gradual reduction	57%
Maintained at current reduced level	26%
Quit	17%

Follow-up studies showed that a substantial proportion of smokers attending the workshop were successful in maintaining their patterns of controlled smoking.[5]

Controlling Your Puffing Patterns

The controlled smoking described above encouraged health-concerned smokers to reduce their smoke intake by paying special attention to three factors: the brand of cigarette smoked, the number of cigarettes smoked per day, and the amount of each cigarette actually smoked. But as other researchers have pointed out, a health-concerned smoker who wishes to cut down can modify a number of other factors as well:[6]

- Puff frequency—the number of times a lit cigarette comes in contact with the smoker's lips.
- Puff length—the amount of time during which the smoker draws air through the cigarette on each puff.
- Depth of inhalation—the amount of smoke drawn into the lungs with each puff.
- Inter-puff interval—the time between one puff and the next.
- Cigarette duration—the time between lighting and extinguishing a cigarette.

Increased awareness and control of puffing patterns may be a necessary step in attaining some of the proposed benefits of switching to low-tar cigarettes. When smokers switch to a low-tar brand, there *is* a risk of compensating by taking deeper and more frequent drags (see chapter 7), but even if they do compensate somewhat, smokers who switch brands and reduce the number of cigarettes smoked may still benefit from cutting down. And decreasing one's exposure to tobacco smoke can be the beginning of a gradual process that eventually leads to quitting.[7]

Two-step Inhaling

Studies suggest that smokers who do not inhale are at considerably lower health risk than smokers who inhale moderately or deeply.[8]

Degree of Inhalation	Relative Death Rate
Never smoked	1.00
Do not inhale	1.33
Inhale slightly	1.53
Inhale moderately	1.81
Inhale deeply	2.21

For smokers who do inhale, the pattern of inhalation may have a considerable influence on the way the inhaled smoke affects the lungs. Two-step inhaling—drawing smoke first into the mouth, diluting it with air, then breathing in the diluted smoke—appears less likely to trigger the so-called acute airway response observed in smokers who draw smoke directly into their lungs. In the acute airway response, the airways leading to the lungs narrow for a few seconds. As one smoking researcher observed: "The manner of smoke inhalation affects the relative concentrations of the different constituents reaching the lungs and also appears to be the main determinant of the acute airway response to smoking, which was unrelated to the number of cigarettes smoked or the tar content of the smoke. This suggests that patterns of smoke inhalation may influence the pathogenesis of bronchial disease associated with smoking."[9]

Training Yourself to Smoke Less

Barbara Stephens Brockway and her colleagues at the University of Wisconsin at Madison did a study in which they successfully taught smokers to control their smoking behavior.

They began by asking the subjects in their study to answer the following questions for each cigarette they smoked for five consecutive days:

- What time did you light up?
- Were you alone or with others?
- What were you doing?
- How were you feeling?
- How strong was your desire to smoke?

They then asked their subjects to name eight categories of smoking situations that they most frequently encountered. They were asked to rank the situations in which they had the least desire to smoke first, and those in which they had the greatest desire to smoke last. Here is one student's list:

1. Driving a car and/or waiting for people.
2. Sitting in class.
3. Talking on the telephone.
4. Attending business meetings.
5. Sitting at my desk at work.
6. After meals or with coffee.
7. In any relaxed situation (e.g., watching TV or reading).
8. When socializing at parties and/or drinking with friends.

The subjects were then asked to eliminate all cigarettes in each category, beginning with the categories they thought would be easiest. They were also asked to choose alternative behaviors they could adopt when they felt the urge to smoke. The researchers suggested that these alternative behaviors should be unobtrusive and socially acceptable; should be performed for a period of at least five seconds; should be easily accessible in high-anxiety situations (methods that require no special equipment or employ something you will always have on hand—e.g., a paper clip or a pencil); should be limited to one or two standard responses per person; and should not involve putting anything into the mouth.

Subjects were encouraged to experiment with a number of possible alternative behaviors before narrowing their choice to one or two. Alternative responses actually chosen include the following:

- Taking ten deep, slow, relaxing breaths.
- Bending a paper clip.
- Rubbing a smooth stone kept in a pocket.
- Going for a walk.
- Going through the steps of a memorized relaxation exercise.
- Thinking of three positive effects of not smoking.

The subjects also practiced handling high-risk smoking situations that required assertive behavior—such as what to do if they were offered a cigarette and did not wish to smoke. Subjects also assumed the role of an ex-smoker describing the benefits they had received from ending their smoking habit. The last two sessions of the class were held at a local restaurant and a local bar.

Follow-up studies showed that those who followed the program either quit or continued to smoke at reduced levels for up to six months. However, those who had not quit by twelve months after the class tended to revert to their former smoking patterns. These results confirm Dr. Glasgow's belief that controlled smoking is most effec-

tive when used as a transitional method on the way to
quitting.[10]

Strategic Withdrawal

Researchers Arden Christen and Kenneth Cooper have
proposed that smokers should approach the idea of controlled smoking as the beginning of a long process of
"strategic withdrawal" leading to ultimate quitting:

"Smokers are often an unforgiving lot. They frequently feel that quitting is an all-or-nothing proposition,
and fail to understand the significance of the dose response relationship: the less one smokes, the less the
hazard. The smoker who has gone from three or four
packs a day to one pack a day should realize that he has
made great strides. Many people appear to quit in graduated fashion over a prolonged period, and some have
reported that a tapering-off process is the preferable way
to quit. As Mark Twain said, 'Habit is habit, and not to
be flung out the window by any man, but coaxed down-
stairs a step at a time.' Of the many who have succeeded
in quitting, about 50 percent reported that they stopped
suddenly and 50 percent that they stopped gradually.

"For some, the very *idea* that they could stop smoking
is one that evolves very slowly."[11]

The Time-based Quota Technique

Let's say you want to limit your smoking to 20 cigarettes
per day. If you get up at 7:30 and go to bed at 11:30,
you are awake for 16 hours; 16 hours times 60 min per
hour = 960 minutes; 960 minutes divided by 20 cigarettes per day equals 48 minutes per cigarette. So allow-
ing a minimum of 10 minutes per cigarette, you should

allow no less than 38 minutes from the time you put out one cigarette until you light the next.

Humor writer Alice Kahn, who is also a nurse practitioner, says: "I've been having good results encouraging my clients to begin smoking on a preplanned time schedule. If they are smoking 15 cigarettes per day, I have them write out a complete time schedule for when they will smoke each one—just like any other drug. Then, when they wish, they can begin to withdraw cigarettes from their schedule."[12]

How do you know when it's time for the next cigarette? The easiest way is to wear a wristwatch with a countdown timer. When you finish a cigarette, simply start your timer. And don't light another cigarette until your watch beeps. You can then cut your smoke intake by simply setting your countdown timer for longer and longer intervals.[13] (Also see the LifeSign Quit-Smoking Computer, p. 196.)

The "Part-time Nonsmoker" Technique

In this approach you choose a part of the day during which you would be most comfortable being a non-smoker. This may be first thing in the morning, in the middle of the day, or after a certain hour. You divide your day into "smoking time" and "nonsmoking time." Then you gradually extend your nonsmoking time while cutting down on your smoking time.

Replacing Cigarettes with Substitute Activities

Develop a list of innovative and enjoyable alternative activities, things you can do when you feel the urge to smoke.

- Healthy foods provide an excellent alternative: Munch on carrots, wheat thins, melba toast, sunflower seeds, orange segments, apples, celery, pretzel sticks, half a banana; drink a small glass of orange, tomato, or apple juice.

- Water can be used in a number of ways: You can drink a glass of ice or mineral water, take a shower, take a bath, or go swimming.

- Exercise is always a healthy alternative: Go for a walk around the block, skip rope for five minutes, do yoga exercises or other stretches, or exercise your lungs by breathing in deeply, then exhaling through pursed lips. Repeat 10 times.

Avoiding Smoking Triggers

Every smoker has his or her own key smoking triggers. Watch out for these and avoid them. Common smoking triggers (and some tips for avoiding them) include:

- Talking on the phone. (Stand instead of sitting. Use a phone other than the one you normally use.)

- Having your morning cup of coffee. (Have breakfast in the non-smoking section of your favorite restaurant.)

- When you are hungry. (Drink 6 to 8 glasses of water a day to keep yourself feeling full.)

- With alcoholic beverages. (Cut down on wine, beer, and liquor. Order nonalcoholic beer, wine, or cocktails.)

- After a meal. (Get up immediately after eating and begin an enjoyable nonsmoking activity.)

- Use the acronym HALT to help you remember to avoid what may be the four biggest smoking triggers of all—situations in which you are *H*ungry, *A*ngry, *L*onely, or *T*ired.

Controlled Smoking: Variations

An extreme but potentially effective alternative approach to controlled smoking is the Miller Method, developed by psychologist Richard Miller of California's Wilbur Hot Springs Health Sanctuary. Miller advised health-concerned smokers to smoke as many cigarettes as they wish per day *but to take only one puff on each cigarette,* then put it out. Miller acknowledges that his method has never been subjected to scientific study, but says that in his experience, every person who has followed these directions to the letter has stopped smoking within a few days or weeks.[14]

Another variation of the controlled smoking approach is the Kern Method, developed by computer operator Alan Kern. Kern felt that it would be easier to count the number of *puffs* he took than to measure each cigarette he smoked.

To use the Kern Method, observe your average number of puffs. Let's say you average 12 puffs per cigarette. For each cigarette you smoke this week, limit yourself to 11 puffs. The next week, limit yourself to 10 puffs. The week after, 9, and so on.

Be sure you don't increase the length and depth of your puffs. In a little over three months, you'll be down to one puff per cigarette. Maintain this level until you're ready to quit.

More Tips for Cutting Down

- Stop buying cartons—buy only single packs

- Smoke the last cigarette in one pack before buying the next.

- Stop carrying cigarettes. Leave them in inconvenient places.

- Make your house off-limits for smoking. Go outside to smoke.

- Chew gum, candy, licorice sticks, toothpicks, carrots, celery.

- Record your number of cigarettes smoked each day and display this number prominently on your refrigerator.

- Get in the habit of taking a shower or hot bath at the times you would normally have your "most important" cigarettes.

- Increase your level of physical activity.

- Keep a "butt bottle" in each of the places you are accustomed to smoke. (A gallon jug works nicely.) Use it as your ashtray. Drop all extinguished cigarettes into your butt bottle. Keep it in plain view. Do *not* empty your butt bottle. If it fills up, start another one. Continue to keep your butt bottle(s) in plain view until you finally quit.

7

Cutting Your Risk by Switching Brands

English smoking researcher M.A.H. Russell has written: "It is unlikely that any single measure has saved more lives or done more to reduce smoking-related disease than the switch from plain to filter-tipped cigarettes." In 1955, less than 2 percent of all cigarettes smoked had filters. By 1975, that figure had increased to over 84 percent. By 1984, 92 percent of all cigarettes sold had filter tips.[1]

It is no overstatement to say that over the past two decades, the American cigarette has been almost totally transformed.[2] Over this period the tobacco industry has changed its methods of cultivating, processing, and curing tobacco. Ironically enough, some researchers speculate that some of the pesticides, herbicides, and fertilizers used today may make tobacco even more dangerous than it was "back in the good old days."

In addition to dozens of new types of filters, the tobacco industry has added the following innovations:

- Filter additives.
- Vents for adding air to inhaled smoke.

- High-porosity paper to dilute inhaled smoke.
- Tobacco additives that lower combustion temperatures.
- Papers that burn faster and thus reduce the time a cigarette burns.

Many of these changes have come in response to increasing consumer demand for low-tar cigarettes. There has also been substantial support from federal policymakers: The National Cancer Institute alone has spent over $40 million to help develop less hazardous cigarettes.

The response of health-conscious consumers to low-tar brands has been extraordinary. The low-tar share of the cigarette market in the United States tripled between 1976 and 1982. A similar pattern has been observed in Canada. These changes have been greatest among women, whites, the well-educated, and the more affluent.[3]

Filters vs. Nonfilters: Are They Safer?

Studies show that cigarette filters *do* partially reduce a smoker's risk of lung cancer and cancer of the larynx. The cancer rates of smokers of filter and nonfilter cigarettes are shown in the graph below:

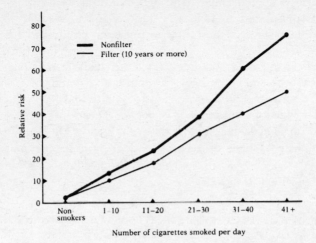

Figure 7-1 Lung Cancer Rates for Smokers of Filtered and Unfiltered Cigarettes[4]

However, it appears that cigarette filters alone produce little or no reduction in smokers' risk of heart disease. This is presumably because the constituent of tobacco smoke that has the most adverse effect on the heart is carbon monoxide, and no filter to date has been able to remove carbon monoxide from tobacco smoke.[5]

Switching to Low-tar Cigarettes

Unless they carefully follow a program (such as the program of controlled smoking described in the previous chapter), most smokers who switch to low-tar cigarettes unconsciously alter their puffing patterns and number of cigarettes smoked so as to take in a level of nicotine only slightly below former levels. In some cases this may actually lead to an *increased* intake of carbon monoxide.[6]

There *is* some benefit in switching brands, however, and this seems to hold true even if the new brand is smoked in an uncontrolled manner. In addition to the decreased risk of lung cancer, those who switch to low-tar, low-nicotine cigarettes are more likely to quit than those who smoke medium- or high-dose cigarettes.[7]

Health-concerned smokers who want to make substantial reductions in both lung cancer *and* heart disease risk can do so by switching to a lower-tar brand while following the guidelines for controlled smoking in the previous chapter. Of course, the greatest risk reduction of all can be obtained from quitting.

FTC Tar and Nicotine Tables: How Reliable?

The Federal Trade Commission issues tables listing the tar, nicotine, and carbon monoxide content of all U.S. cigarettes. (The current version of this table is reproduced in Appendix IV; see page 273.) But the data in this table should be taken with a grain of salt, since the levels listed may not correspond to the results smokers actually obtain. This is because these values are calculated by using smoking machines.

Most smoking machines are set to take a 35-ml. two-second puff once per minute. Unlike machines, however, human smokers vary tremendously in their smoking habits. Studies show that the average smoker takes a puff of 2.5 to 3 seconds duration every 45 to 50 seconds (women inhale slightly more frequently than men). Smokers can—and do—vary their smoking behavior in a variety of ways that influence the amount of tobacco smoke to which they are exposed. Some take much larger or much smaller puffs, and many vary the frequency of their puffs. One smoker might take a 1-second puff every 3 minutes, while another might take a 7-second puff every 30 seconds. As a result, two smokers smoking identical cigarettes can have a tenfold or even one hundredfold difference in tars and carbon monoxide actually consumed.[8]

This wide variation led one smoking researcher to conclude: "The range of constituent levels for a single cigarette brand is greater than the range recorded for all 115 cigarette brands tested."[9]

Let's look at a hypothetical example:

You're at a party. Two different people ask you if they can bum a cigarette. You give each of them one of your low-tar, low-nicotine cigarettes, which are rated at 0.4 mg. of tar.

Harvey Hacker is a three-pack-a-day smoker who has run out of his own high-tar brand. He seems to suck the very life out of the cigarette. He takes huge drags, one after another, drawing the smoke directly into his lungs, then holding it in as long as possible. He squeezes the filter tightly, blocking the vent holes. He smokes the cigarette all the way down to the filter. Harvey may take in as much as 8 to 10 mg. of tar from this so-called low-tar cigarette.

Minnie Minimal bums an identical cigarette. But Minnie is a minimal smoker. She never smokes more than one or two cigarettes a week—usually at parties, while having a drink. She enjoys holding it, playing with it, and watching the smoke, but she has never inhaled. In fact, several full inhales would probably make her dizzy. She absorbs a bit of smoke through the lining of her mouth and nose, and may inadvertently breathe in a tiny bit. Her final intake is 1/10 of a milligram—roughly 1/100 the dose taken in by Harvey.

"Cheating" on FTC Tar Tests

As if things were not already confused enough, the Federal Trade Commission has charged certain cigarette manufacturers with "cheating" on FTC tar and nicotine tests by designing filters that will deliver very low tar levels when smoked on a smoking machine but much higher levels when smoked by actual smokers. For example, the FTC claims that the effective tar rating for one brand of cigarettes, officially listed at 1.0 mg., should be three to seven times as high.[10]

How Smokers Compensate for Low-Tar Cigarettes

What do smokers do to obtain increased amounts of nicotine (and other toxic substances) from low-tar cigarettes? They take more puffs per cigarette; take in more smoke per puff; inhale directly rather than in a two-step process; inhale more deeply; hold the smoke in longer; and block the air holes in the filter.

One study found that blocking the air channels in a cigarette filter could increase the tar content of smoke by 51 percent while increasing carbon monoxide content by 147 percent. And of smokers who smoke cigarettes with vented filters, studies show that 95 percent block the vent hole with their fingers. This is particularly common during the last few puffs, when it is difficult to grasp the cigarette without blocking the air vents. Researchers advise that the only foolproof way to keep from blocking the air vents is to use a cigarette holder. Some holders allow smokers to further decrease the amount of tar and carbon monoxide in each puff by adding additional air to the stream of tobacco smoke.[11]

The Phaseout Alternative

Another way to decrease the dose of toxic materials you receive from each puff is by using a device about the size of a cigarette pack to make tiny holes in the filter ends of your cigarettes. These pinholes allow cool air from outside the cigarette to mix with the tobacco smoke, thus diluting the smoke and decreasing the level of tar, carbon monoxide, and other toxic gases which reach the smoker's lungs.

To use the device (brand name: Phaseout) the smoker inserts the filter end of an unopened pack of cigarettes into a slot in the unit and then presses down on a lever which drives a row of long needles through the pack. By repositioning the pack and resetting the machine, the smoker can make one, two, three, or four holes in each cigarette. The greater the number of holes, the greater the reduction of tar and carbon monoxide. The manufacturer claims that smokers who use the device can reduce their tar and carbon monoxide by as much as 90 percent—without changing brands.

The unit is endorsed by the World Organization for Science and Health and comes with instructions for gradually reducing the concentration of toxic substances in your present brand over a period of eight weeks. The Phaseout costs about $25. It can be ordered from Products & Patents Ltd., 140 Broadway, Lynbrook, NY 11563, (516) 599-1900.

Self-Testing for Tar Intake

Here are two ways to check on how much tar you're really getting:

- Look at the filter on the cigarette you're smoking.

If you are *not* blocking the air holes, you'll see a small area of brownish stain in the center of the filter. This small, circular stain will be surrounded by an outer ring of white, unstained filter. If the outer part of the filter is stained with tar, it means that you *are* blocking the filter holes. (Due to their different design, this test may not work with Barclay, Kool Ultra, and some other brands.)

- Look at the filter on a cigarette you've already smoked. How dark is the stain? The darker it is, the more tar you're getting. See if you can find ways to smoke that will result in less stain on the filter. The cleaner the filter, the cleaner your lungs.[12]

If You Switch to a Low-tar Brand: Avoiding Nicotine Compensation

Some smokers compensate so much that they are able to obtain the same nicotine levels they reached with their former high-tar brand. Others are able to make such a switch with only minor compensation. Studies suggest that a smoker's level of compensation varies from day to day and from moment to moment.

It *is* possible to switch brands *without* increasing one's dose of tobacco smoke per cigarette, but to do so, smokers who inhale must practice controlled smoking—that is, they must not increase either the *number* of cigarettes smoked or the *portion* of each cigarette smoked, and they must not change their puffing pattern so as to take in more smoke per puff.[13] Guidelines for controlled smoking are listed in chapter 6.

Cigars and Pipes: Are They Safer?

Some studies show that pipe and cigar smokers have substantially lower death rates than cigarette smokers. The classic 1958 study by Hammond and Horn found that while death rates were increased by 68 percent among men who smoked cigarettes, they were increased by only 12 percent among men who smoked cigars, and by 9 percent in men who smoked pipes.[14]

One might think such statistics would be enough to send cigarette smokers running down to their local pipe and cigar shop. Unfortunately, it may not be all that easy. Most smoking researchers *discourage* cigarette smokers from switching to pipes or cigars, because unlike so-called "primary" pipe or cigar smokers (those who have never smoked cigarettes) who inhale little or no smoke, former cigarette smokers who switch to pipes or cigars ("secondary" pipe and cigar smokers) tend to continue to inhale high doses of tobacco smoke. If they do, they are likely to have carbon monoxide blood levels equivalent to those of persons who have never been anything but cigarette smokers. However, secondary pipe and cigar smokers may succeed in reducing their intake of tar: Research suggests that when either cigarette tobacco or pipe tobacco is smoked in a pipe, there is a substantial reduction—approximately tenfold—in the concentration of particulate matter in the inhaled smoke. Pipes that contain more elaborate filters may produce an even greater reduction.[15].

A recent European study found that the relative risk of lung cancer for the following groups of smokers was as follows:[16]

Nonsmokers	1.1
Pipe only	2.5
Cigar only	2.9

Cigarette and cigar	6.9
Cigarette and pipe	8.1
Cigarette only	9.0

PIPE GUIDELINES

Cigarette smokers who wish to switch to a pipe can substantially reduce their risk—provided they follow the following guidelines:

- Draw lightly on the bowl.

- Don't inhale. Pipe smokers who do not inhale are at only slightly increased risk for heart disease and lung cancer. However, they have just as high a risk of cancer of the mouth, esophagus, and larynx as cigarette smokers.

- Smoke a pipe with a filter. This will help reduce the tiny airborne particles in the smoke.

- Gradually cut down on the number of times per day you smoke your pipe.

CIGAR GUIDELINES

Many of the guidelines for smoking pipes can be applied to cigars as well. Primary cigar smokers (those who have never been regular cigarette smokers) generally don't inhale. Thus, they have fairly low health risks. But cigarette smokers who switch to cigars usually continue to inhale after they switch to cigars—in many cases without even realizing they're doing so. A Florida study suggests that inhaling cigar smoke may be *much worse* than inhaling cigarette smoke. It found that cigar smokers who inhale had substantially higher blood carbon monoxide levels than cigarette smokers. So switching to cigars is not recommended unless you are positive that you can do so without inhaling.[17]

Smokers who presently smoke cigars should follow these guidelines:

- Don't inhale.
- Smoke as few cigars as possible.
- Switch to smaller, milder brands.

Snuff and Chewing Tobacco

Many people think that chewing tobacco and snuff went out with the handlebar mustache and the celluloid collar. Unfortunately, this is not the case. The use of these oral tobacco products has been growing rapidly in recent years, particularly among teenage and young adult males. An estimated 12 million people used smokeless tobacco in the U.S. in 1985. About half of these used it regularly. A 1986 report to the Surgeon General found that 16 percent of U.S. males between the ages of twelve and twenty-five had used smokeless tobacco within the previous year. In many parts of the country, as many as 25 to 35 percent of adolescent males use smokeless tobacco.

Many users believe that chewing tobacco is not harmful. But a recent Surgeon General's report concluded that smokeless tobacco "represents a significant health risk. It is not a safe substitute for smoking cigarettes. It can cause cancer and a number of noncancerous oral conditions and can lead to nicotine addiction and dependence."

Recent studies link chewing tobacco to an increased risk of cancer of the mouth, cheek, gum, tongue, and palate. And because it contains more nicotine, chewing tobacco may actually be even more highly addictive than smoking cigarettes. For cigarette smokers who *also* chew tobacco, these risks are considerably higher. Because of its high salt content, smokeless tobacco has also been implicated as an aggravating factor in high blood pressure.

The Cigarette of the Future

Researchers are continuing to develop ways of making cigarettes even safer. Here are some of the strategies currently in the development stage:

- A filter that becomes more active as the cigarette burns farther down.[18]

- A biological filter that uses green algae to denature toxic substances. Unlike other filters, the algae filter is able to trap and denature carbon monoxide.[19]

- A cigarette made with high-selenium tobacco. Studies suggest that rates of lung cancer for smokers are significantly lower in countries with selenium-rich soils. One team of researchers concluded: ''It is possible that relatively high selenium concentrations in tobaccos could aid in modifying cigarette smoke-induced carcinogenesis by interacting directly with carcinogens in the particulate or gas phases of smoke.''[20]

- Low polonium 210 cigarettes. There is some evidence to suggest that lung cancer in smokers is caused by the radioactive element polonium 210. It is the only component of cigarette smoke that has produced tumors, by itself, when inhaled by laboratory animals. Smokers have about three times as much polonium 210 in their lungs as nonsmokers. Certain varieties of tobacco accumulate substantially less of this element. Polonium 210 levels can also be decreased by appropriate choices of soil and fertilizer, by spacing the plants closer together, and by the use of chemical agents.[21]

- Cigarettes that contain nicotine but no tobacco. Nicotine-containing placebo cigarettes may turn out to be the most exciting breakthrough since the filter tip, though some questions still remain about this very promising product. (For more on nicotine-containing placebo cigarettes, see chapter 9.)

8

Getting Ready to Quit: What You Need to Know

One of the biggest mistakes potential quitters make is trying to quit without proper preparation. The successful ex-smokers we spoke with advised that the period of getting ready to quit may well be the most important time of all.[1]

How long this period lasts depends on how well prepared you are right now. Most of the successful quitters we interviewed told us it took them several months from the time they first seriously decided they would quit to the time when they actually succeeded in doing so. Remember, quitting is a long-term process. Don't be in too much of a hurry. You should strive for gradual, steady progress toward your goal.

A Million Successful Quitters Per Year

It's encouraging to realize that in quitting you'll be taking part in a massive social movement. For the past twenty years, more than a million people per year have quit smoking in the U.S. alone.[2]

These new ex-smokers are a sophisticated bunch. They know that quitting is not a simple process. It is not merely a matter of willpower. Rather, it is a matter of acquiring and practicing a variety of skills that will increase your awareness of your own behavior and give you a greater degree of control over it.

Perhaps even more important, successful quitting will require profound changes in your thinking. It will affect every level of your daily activities and social interactions. For many smokers, especially those who smoke only a few cigarettes per day, quitting may be relatively easy. For heavier smokers, it may not be easy, but it *is* possible.

Above all, successful quitters emphasize that *quitting is something you have to do for yourself.* Many smokers fail to quit because they expect to find an expert, a drug, a device, or other outside power to magically make them ex-smokers.

You will have some very powerful tools on your side. Books like this one can be a great help. Physicians or other experts can offer invaluable advice. Nicotine gum can help ease you through the withdrawal process. Supportive friends can make a tremendous difference. But no tool, drug, expert, or friend can do it for you. The successful quitters we interviewed all said that to succeed you have to accept the fact that the final responsibility for quitting is your own.

Quitting on Your Own

The fact is that most smokers who have given up cigarettes have done so *without involvement in any formal
program,* although many of these successful quitters have
used books, tapes, or other sources of expert advice.[3]

"An estimated 40 million people have given up smoking on their own," says Frank Riessman, Director of
New York's National Self-Help Clearinghouse. "They
have accomplished this goal without joining any group
or engaging in any formal program. These successful
quitters have developed their own plan for quitting, have
put that plan into action, and have succeeded in becoming ex-smokers. And if 40 million people have done it,
so can you."[4]

Indeed, although programs run by therapists can be
helpful adjuncts to a person's own quitting plan, even
those smokers who make use of such groups should not
expect the program to "do it for them." According to
Jackie C. Wood, Ph.D., of the Stanford Medical Group,
Stanford University Medical Center, "The more therapist-
intensive the method, that is, the more that is done for
the smoker relative to what the smoker does for himself,
the higher the probability of relapse."[5]

Many smokers feel pessimistic about quitting. And
some studies do seem to bear out such pessimism. But
virtually all such studies look only at a *single* attempt to
quit. Thus, much of the available evidence may overstate
the difficulty of the task. Most short-term studies show
success rates of roughly 20 to 30 percent.[6] But studies
by Columbia University psychologist and smoking researcher Stanley Schachter, Ph.D., show that 64 percent
of the smokers who tried to quit on their own had succeeded. Schachter concludes: "It appears that the generally accepted professional and public impression that

nicotine addiction is an almost hopelessly difficult condition to correct is flatly wrong. People can and do cure themselves of smoking. They do so in large numbers and for long periods of time, and in many cases, apparently, they're able to do so permanently.''[7]

The Ten Stages of Quitting

Smokers tend to think of quitting as a huge, insurmountable obstacle. It's more realistic—and more useful—to think of it as a gradual, step-by-step process that may last for months or even years.

Here is what to expect along the way:

- Stage One—You have identified yourself as a health-concerned smoker. You are worried about the effects of smoking on your health and wonder if you should quit or cut down.

- Stage Two—You decide that you will seek additional information about smoking and quitting and begin to actively explore your alternatives.

- Stage Three—You decide to take some steps to modify your smoking level and/or overall health status—switching brands, cutting down, getting more exercise, taking vitamins, managing stressful situations more effectively, paying more attention to your bonds with friends and family, etc.

- Stage Four—You make a firm commitment to quit but do not specify a quitting date.

- Stage Five—You set a quitting date and make a firm commitment to quit on that date.

- Stage Six—You smoke your last cigarette and go without smoking for 24 hours.

- Stage Seven—You complete your first week as a nonsmoker.

- Stage Eight—You complete your first month as as nonsmoker.

- Stage Nine—You complete your first three months as a nonsmoker.

- Stage Ten—You complete your first year as a nonsmoker.

Note: A table of suggested activities for each of these ten stages appears at the end of this chapter.

You may already have come a good part of the way toward your goal. The very fact that you are reading this book suggests that you have already reached at least stage two of the quitting process.

It is important for aspiring quitters to realize that during stages one through five, they may find themselves in a state of profound and confusing ambivalence. Studies show that during this period a smoker's *positive* feelings about smoking do not disappear, although their *negative* feelings increase considerably. Thus a smoker preparing to quit may experience violently opposing feelings about his or her smoking habit.

It is only after smokers actually quit that this conflict begins to ease. New ex-smokers gradually lose their positive feelings about cigarettes, and the conflict diminishes.

Here's a useful exercise for potential quitters suggested by smoking researcher Saul Shiffman. At several times during the process of quitting, make a list of the pros and cons of smoking. Chances are that in stages one through five, they will be fairly evenly balanced. But after you have actually quit, you'll see that the list of cons gets longer while the list of pros gets shorter and shorter—and gradually disappears altogether.[9]

Reasons to Quit

This exercise was inspired by the Willie Nelson song of the same name. Here's what you do:

Buy a packet of 100 3 × 5 index cards. Write a *reason to quit* on each card. Examples: "Smoking makes me short of breath." "Smoking makes my clothes smell bad." "Smoking is a sexual turn-off for your mate." "Smoking is bad for my daughter." "Smoking is literally rotting my lungs." "Smoking is a dirty, stupid habit."

Make at least three to five new cards per day. Be sure to include the specific effects of smoking on your health—shortness of breath, a morning cough, sore throats, wrinkled skin, or any negative effects on your sex drive. Keep it up until you have written down at least 100 reasons to quit. Carry your cards with you at all times and review them regularly. Read your remarks aloud to friends. Continue to make up new ones as you think of additional reasons to quit.

Once you have accumulated a substantial number of these cards, reread the reason for quitting on the front, then, on the back, write a corresponding *benefit* you will receive as a nonsmoker. Example: If you wrote on the front of one of your cards, "My health is much worse because I smoke," you might write on the back: "As a nonsmoker, I will experience a dramatic increase in my health over the first few months after I quit."

If you wrote, "Smoking makes me very critical of myself. It makes me doubt my ability to control my own life," you might write on the back: "As a nonsmoker, I will no longer be so self-critical. I will know that I am truly in control of my life.''

Review the pros and cons frequently and continue to add to them. Use your cards until you reach stage ten of the quitting process.

Developing Your Own Quitting Plan

An absolute must: *Don't try to quit before you feel ready.* Give yourself the time you need to build up your commitment, set up your social support system, and learn new skills that will help you succeed when you reach the quitting date you have selected.

Be patient. Most successful quitters go through a long period of building commitment and increasing their awareness, tapering down, and learning new coping skills before they finally quit.

Identify and combine the methods you think will work best for you. Give yourself time and permission to develop your own, personalized way to quit. Each of the successful quitters we interviewed told us that they had gone through an intense period of consciousness-raising both before and during their efforts to quit. Researchers at the University of Missouri have found that successful quitters tend to use a greater variety of coping strategies than those who do not succeed.[10]

In forming your plan, emphasize strategies that will add value, meaning, and enjoyment to your life. Emphasize the things you *want* to do, and keep the number of things you think you *should* do to an absolute minimum. According to Jackie C. Wood of the Stanford Medical Group, ''When 'shoulds' predominate, the ex-smoker feels out of control and relapse is likely.'' Dr. Wood advises that smokers can increase their chance of success by replacing smoking with such ''positive addictions'' as physical exercise, meditation, healthy social activities, and enjoyable hobbies.[11]

Do all you can to reduce the stress in your life. High levels of stress are one of the most common reasons for failure.[12] Smoking researchers and successful ex-smokers agree in warning health-concerned smokers *not* to set a quitting date that occurs at a particularly high-stress time—moving, changing jobs, major deadlines, ending or beginning a serious relationship. You can increase your chances of success by choosing a quitting date that will be followed by a relatively stable period of at least four weeks.

A team of Harvard researchers found that successful quitters exhibited the following characteristics during their pre-quitting phase:

- high expectations of success;
- fewer cigarettes per day;
- low level of stress;
- high degree of personal security and self-confidence.

There is every indication that those whose patterns approximate these can improve their chances of succeeding.[13]

How do you know when you're ready to quit? There is no simple answer to this question, but the best advice seems to be to wait until you feel extremely confident of success. Many studies have concluded that the single most important predictor of successful quitting is the smoker's degree of confidence that he or she *will* succeed. Study after study shows that the smokers who were most strongly convinced of their ability to succeed were indeed most successful. As one researcher wrote, "Belief in success was a necessary precursor to actual success." Such studies suggest that health-concerned smokers would be well advised not to set a quitting date until they feel that the time is really "ripe" for them to quit.[14]

Good Times To Quit

Pick as hassle-free a time as possible. Do all you can to make your first month (and especially your first week) as a nonsmoker as calm as possible. Researchers at St. Louis's Washington University found that smokers who were able to quit during a time when their life was relatively free of problems were much more likely to maintain their nonsmoking status.[15]

Jerome Jaffe, Director of the National Institute of Drug Abuse Addiction Research Center in Baltimore, agrees: "If you're a writer, don't try to quit when you're on a deadline. If you're a tax accountant, don't give it up around April 15. Pick a time when you're less vulnerable."[16]

Quit when you have plenty of energy and attention to devote to getting through your first weeks and months without tobacco. As one successful quitter told us, "A person who is quitting should have only one focus, especially for that first week: getting through the day, each day, without smoking. I found it useful to plan one symbolic activity for each day: planting a tree, buying a new coffee cup, getting my teeth cleaned—each one of them representing a symbolic turning point."

Saul Shiffman concurs. "The whole issue of setting aside time, energy, and attention to quitting smoking is *extremely* important. All too often, people think of quitting smoking as something they can do on the side with one hand tied behind their back. Believe me, it's not that easy. Sometimes when I'm working with a client I'll ask him to imagine that his physician has told him that he must go into the hospital for surgery and must plan to spend a few weeks recuperating. Under such conditions, no one would think it odd to devote a sizable chunk of time and energy to one's health. It is just as important to set aside that time and energy when it comes to quitting."[17]

Look ahead and find—or arrange—a time that will increase your chances of quitting. One successful ex-smoker, a nurse, wrote, "I had tried and failed to quit several times—probably because I attempted to do so during nursing school. It wasn't until after I finished my training, and took a low-stress job in a community hospital, that I was able to quit for good.

"It was an ideal situation for quitting. I had much of my time free for reading, journal keeping, and yoga. I felt particularly good about myself (except for the smoking) and the possibilities for my life ahead. I felt in control of things and really felt up to it."

Other suggestions for picking a quitting date:

- During the American Cancer Society's "Great American Smoke-out." This widely publicized stop-smoking event takes place every year on the Thursday before Thanksgiving.

- On New Year's Day.

- On the first day of April. One ex-smoker commented: "I decided to quit on April Fool's Day— because I felt like such a fool for sucking that junk into my body for all those years."

- On your birthday.

- On the anniversary of a loved one's death.

- After an episode of illness or injury—especially if you have cut down or quit while recuperating.

- When you are ill or have a troublesome smoking-related symptom.

- Following the resolution of some major life difficulty. As one successful ex-smoker told us, "I had just gone through an excruciatingly painful divorce. Several months later, when I was well on the way to recovery, I decided to turn a bad experience into a good one by giving up cigarettes. When I succeeded in staying free from cigarettes for two months, I knew it was all going to be OK."

- On a birthday, holiday, or other significant date as a gift to a friend or family member who especially would like you to quit.

Poor Times to Quit

- High-stress times.

- Immediately after a serious loss or a difficult transition.

- Periods in which you have little contact with friends or family members.

- Immediately after the death of a loved one.

- Just before a holiday. If you're concerned about weight gain, it may be best not to quit when you'd be especially tempted to "pig out" on holiday goodies.

Don't Procrastinate

But as soon as your life circumstances do seem fairly favorable, *go for it*. Set a quitting date within the next two weeks. Here's what smoking researcher Saul Shiffman has to say about the importance of decisive action: "I've just finished a study in which we interviewed people before and after they quit—or failed to quit. Much to my surprise, those who quit at all quit on or very close to their designated quitting date. People who failed to quit by their quit date were very unlikely to quit later. The bottom line seems to be to structure things so that you avoid procrastination and an infinite delay.''[18]

Recognizing Rationalizations

A number of common rationalizations play a large part in inducing successful quitters to begin smoking again, for example:

- ''Just one cigarette certainly won't hurt me.''
- ''I deserve a cigarette.''
- ''I can't take it anymore. This is unbearable.''

These rationalizations are particularly dangerous when presented to you by well-meaning (or not-so-well meaning) friends. It is a worthwhile exercise to think through some of these rationalizations and other high-risk remarks or situations and practice responding to them in a way that supports your resolve to remain a nonsmoker.

Pro-Smoking Argument	*Antismoking Response*[19]
One little cigarette won't hurt you.	No thanks. I am *so* delighted I've been able to quit that I'm not about to give it up for *anything*.
Go on. Be sociable. Have a cigarette.	I'll be glad to keep my friends company, but I don't smoke anymore. I wish they'd quit and keep *me* company.

Come on, you need a ciga-
rette. You've been grouchy as
hell since you quit.

I'm still adjusting to doing
without nicotine. I think I'll
go for a walk. It'll help me
get rid of some of this nervous energy.

Come on. Have a cigarette.
What're you afraid of, anyway?

Not much—just lung cancer,
heart disease, emphysema, diabetes, wrinkled skin, sexual
impotence, bad breath, and
dying before my time.

Keeping a Smoking Journal

A number of successful ex-smokers suggested that a
smoking journal, in which you record your thoughts,
feelings, and observations about smoking, can be a valuable part of a quitting program. You can use your smoking journal to help you put together your quitting plan,
to record your urges to smoke and the number of cigarettes you actually do smoke, and to describe the role
smoking plays in your life. (For a model form to use to
keep track of cigarettes smoked, see the section on
Charting Your Smoking in chapter 10.)

You may also wish to use your notebook to make a list
of key support people you'll want to be involved in your
quitting efforts; to record information on smoking groups,
aids, and resources; and to write out your contract to
quit.

Defusing Your Cigarette Triggers

A cigarette trigger is a situation or a feeling that makes
you want a cigarette. It can be a very useful exercise for
smokers to identify the cigarette triggers in their lives.

By identifying these triggers, smokers become more aware of the difference between the trigger itself (stimulus), the urge that it brings on, and the way they choose to respond to that urge. Once you have identified a cigarette trigger, you can use your new awareness to break the cycle by (1) avoiding the stimulus; (2) modifying the stimulus; (3) modifying the environment to permit other responses (behavioral coping); or by (4) modifying your thinking to permit other responses (cognitive coping).

Let's see how these principles can be put into practice. Shelly, one of our interview subjects, is a successful travel agent. Like most travel agents, she spends several hours a day on the phone.

Shelly used to keep a large ashtray on her desk and a carton of Marlboros in her desk drawer. When she began analyzing her smoking patterns, she realized that her office phone had become a powerful cigarette trigger.

Since it wasn't possible for Shelly to do her job without using the phone, she decided to modify her environment to promote alternative responses. She threw her ashtray away and put a photo of her daughter in its place. Every time she has the urge to light a cigarette while she is on the phone, Shelly looks at her daughter's photo instead.

"I'll pick up a pencil. I hold the phone in my right hand rather than my left. And every day for the first few weeks after I quit, I'd bring a little bowl of raw fruit and vegetables to munch on." Shelly also bought a large memo pad to doodle on. And she replaced the cigarettes in her desk drawer with a collection of jigsaw puzzles she bought in a toy store. This kind of practical behavior modification can play an important role in any attempt to control cigarette triggers.

Recognizing a Relapse Crisis

Here are five of the most powerful—and therefore dangerous—triggers for the smokers we interviewed; they correspond very closely to the common relapse situations described by Shiffman.[20] If you find yourself in any of these situations after you quit, you should realize that you may be facing a potential relapse crisis and should prepare to activate emergency coping responses.

1. Social situations in which alcohol is served, especially if others are smoking.
2. Interpersonal conflicts of any kind.
3. Periods of emotional upset, including boredom or depression, especially if you are alone.
4. Relaxing after a meal.
5. Pressure or frustration at work, especially if you are angry or anxious.

Other common cigarette triggers include: drinking a cup of coffee; driving; talking on the phone; a deadline of any kind; taking a break from work; after sex; feeling tense, bored, unhappy, angry, happy, hungry, lonely, tired, sad, or irritable.

Review the relapse crisis situations that would pose the biggest threat in your own situation. Brainstorm a number of possible coping mechanisms to use with each. Practice visualizing what you will do in each situation. Possible suggestions:

- Leave the situation.
- Chew nicotine gum or regular chewing gum.
- Go for a walk, either alone or with a friend.
- Drink a glass of ice water or iced mineral water.
- Munch on raw vegetables and fruit.
- Listen to the radio or watch TV.
- Brush and floss your teeth.

- Chew on a toothpick.
- Exercise.
- Take a shower or a hot bath.
- Call a friend on the phone.
- Listen to music.
- Play the piano (or other instrument).

It may be best to avoid some relapse crisis situations altogether. Alcohol is especially dangerous, both because it can, in itself, be a strong cigarette trigger for many smokers and because self-control is frequently the first thing to go when you've been drinking.

Getting Friends and Family to Help You Quit

Social support can be an important part of your quitting plan. Studies suggest that in many cases, the presence or absence of social support plays a big part in determining whether a smoker will succeed in quitting. Here are some guidelines for getting your own key people to help:

- Ask selected friends if they would be willing to help in your efforts to quit. If they agree, ask them to read Appendix I of this book: "How to Help a Health-Concerned Smoker."

- Warn them that you may be irritable after you quit, especially during the first week. Ask them to be especially nice to you during this time—to ignore your grumpiness or rudeness and to praise you for your efforts to rid yourself of the smoking habit. Assure them that even though you may appear angry, it will be because of the withdrawal process. Assure them too that no matter how you behave, you will need—and appreciate—their help during this time.

• Don't be vague. When friends and family members ask what they can do to help, make specific suggestions. For example:

—"I'd like to be able to call you at any time for the first month after I quit."
—"I'd like you to call me every day for the first three weeks to see how I'm doing."
—"I'd like you to agree to donate X dollars to my health bank if I can stay off cigarettes for a month."
—"I'd like you to invite me to dinner every Wednesday night for the first six weeks after I quit."
—"I'd like you to take the kids for me on Saturday mornings so I can go running."

Ask your smoking support people to observe the following guidelines:[21]

• Praise you for any and all pro-health efforts.
• Reassure you that your efforts to quit will be successful.
• Inquire regularly about how your efforts are proceeding.
• Assure you that the longer you can go without smoking, the easier it will get.
• Ask them not to smoke in your presence.
• Ask them *not* to offer you cigarettes.

GETTING YOUR SPOUSE TO HELP

The role of the spouse seems to be particularly important in quitting. Three University of Oregon researchers who evaluated the spouse's role found that *the spouses of successful quitters were more likely to be cooperative and supportive and less likely to be punishing and controlling* than the spouses of smokers who failed in their efforts to quit. Other studies have concluded that the presence or absence of a supportive spouse is the single most important factor in determining whether a prospective quitter succeeds.

Be sure to warn your spouse that you may become grumpy and irritable after you quit. (One recent quitter described herself as "halfway between an angry old bear and an ornery crab" during her quitting period.) Ask them to simply ignore any obnoxious behavior on your part. Ask them for permission to be as grouchy as you need to be during this time. Assure them that this is just a temporary phase that will pass as your body becomes accustomed to being nicotine-free. Ask them to assure you that they will still love you, no matter how grumpy you become during the first few weeks as a nonsmoker.[22]

USING THE BUDDY SYSTEM

Research shows that prospective quitters who use the buddy system do much better than those who quit on their own. Yale psychologist Irving Janis observed that some members of his smoking cessation groups spontaneously formed "buddy" relationships with others in the group. These pairs of buddies were much more likely to succeed in quitting.

Intrigued by these observations, Janis set up another experiment in which he encouraged group members to form close, high-contact buddy relationships with other group members. A control group received no such instructions. A third group was encouraged to form low-contact buddy type bonds. He then followed the three groups for ten years.

At the end of ten years, the daily smoking consumption of the high-contact buddy pairs was considerably less than that of the smoking level of the control group.[23]

What did these buddies do that was so effective in helping each other quit? They praised each other's successes and criticized each other for backsliding. They supported

each other's desire to quit but refused to accept excuses
for lack of improvement. And they remained in contact
for some time after the end of the formal program.[24]

Going Public or Staying Private

Saul Shiffman advises that publicly announcing one's intention to quit is nearly always helpful. Most smoking
researchers agree. But even so, some smokers take just
the opposite tack—they keep their intentions to themselves. One physician who recently quit recalls: "I didn't
share my quitting with anyone until I was positive I was
going to be successful. However, I'm not sure that was
a good thing. It might have helped. I think I kept it to
myself because I needed to minimize my fear of failure."

If you *do* decide to go public with your plans to quit,
think carefully about whom you will tell. While many of
your friends—particularly nonsmokers—will probably be
quite helpful and supportive, those who smoke may find
the news upsetting. Some may even do their best to discourage you.

But even if some family members and friends offer little or no support, don't lose heart. Studies show that you
can quit anyway. You will simply need to put more em-
phasis on the other tools and techniques at your disposal.
A recent study published in the *Journal of Addictive Behaviors* found that even smokers who had *no* special support for quitting were able to succeed if they were
strongly determined to do so.[25]

Using a Physician or Other Professional

One of the most frequently overlooked resources for smokers determined to quit is a personal physician. Research by Dr. David P. Sachs, a professor at the Stanford School of Medicine, suggests that 60 to 120 seconds of firm, unequivocal, clear-cut medical advice to stop smoking can significantly increase a smoker's chances of quitting. When appropriate, such advice can be supplemented with a prescription for nicotine gum or a referral to a local smoking cessation program.[26]

When you go for your appointment, ask your doctor to explain the principles of nicotine dependence and to share any striking personal anecdotes about patients who contracted smoking-related diseases. Your doctor may be able to arrange for you to visit patients whose smoking contributed to their lung cancer, heart attack, or emphysema. You may also wish to ask your doctor to write you a "prescription" to stop smoking on your chosen quitting date. You may wish to tape the prescription to your refrigerator or put it on your desk until you have been smoke free for 100 days. If you have decided to try nicotine gum, request a prescription from your doctor and ask him to review the instructions for using it.

In addition, you may wish to ask your doctor to write a letter to your employer, requesting that you be granted sick leave to attend smoking cessation groups or clinics. You may also be able to arrange a reduced work load or to take vacation or leave time the week after your quitting date.

In addition to, or instead of, a physician, you may prefer to consult another health professional or counselor (clergy member, psychologist, nurse, physician's assistant, health educator, dentist, physical therapist, chiropractor) or other professional or nonprofessional resources. If so, adapt the above guidelines accordingly. Remember, however, that only a physician or a dentist can give you a prescription for nicotine gum.

Regular Physical Activity

Many successful ex-smokers told us that starting a regular exercise program was an essential part of their own quitting plan. Studies show that regular exercise really *does* increase your chances of quitting. According to one team of smoking researchers, the great majority of smokers who begin to exercise regularly end up quitting, and the higher the level of exercise, the more likely they are to quit. They conclude that it is quite difficult to find even a half-serious regular exerciser who smokes.[27]

One of the best ways to work regular exercise into your daily routine is to find an exercise buddy, someone who wants to take up the same activity you do and is at roughly the same level of fitness and skill. Making appointments with an exercise buddy can be a big help in getting into the habit of doing regular exercise. If you plan to wait and exercise "when you find the time," it will probably never happen. Build exercise into your regular routine. Most regular exercisers schedule their workout during one of three times: first thing in the morning, at lunchtime, or in the early evening, right after work.

Other ideas for building exercise into your routine:

- Parking several blocks away from your office and walking the rest of the way to work (or hopping off the train or bus in advance of your destination).

- Walking instead of driving when errands are within two miles of home.

- Going for a walk after dinner.

- Pedaling an exercise bike while watching the news.

- Signing up for an exercise class or joining a health club.

For additional guidelines on exercise, see chapter 6.

The "Last Exercise"

The following is an extremely effective exercise you can use to provide you with a big burst of motivation as you take the final step and quit cigarettes forever. This approach is adapted from a similar role-playing exercise developed by Yale psychologists Irving Janis and Leon Mann, who found that this type of exercise can be a very powerful factor in making smokers acutely aware of their smoking-related health risks.

In this exercise, you will play the part of a smoker receiving a diagnosis of lung cancer from a physician. We suggest that you do the exercise just before your scheduled quitting date. You can either write your responses in your smoking journal or get one of your smoking support people to play the other parts and act it out like a play.

Here are the directions for the Last Exercise:

- Imagine that you have a cough that refuses to go away. Over the weeks and months it has become such a bother that you have finally consulted a physician. During a previous visit you received a complete physical examination that included X rays and sputum tests. You have now returned to the doctor's office for the final verdict.

- SCENE 1: In the waiting room. Express your thoughts and worries as you wait to see the doctor.
- SCENE 2: Conversation with the physician. The doctor tells you that a definite diagnosis has now been made, and that the news is not good. You have a large malignant mass in your right lung. An operation is needed immediately. You will have to enter the hospital today. Unfortunately, there is only a slight chance that your disease can be cured.
- SCENE 3: The physician steps into another office to arrange for your immediate admission to the hospital. The doctor also arranges for your lawyer to meet you in the hospital so that you can make your last will and testament. Express your thoughts and feelings as you listen to your doctor arranging for your surgery and telling your lawyer about the gravity of the situation. What do you think will happen?
- SCENE 4: Conversation with the physician about the causes of lung cancer. The physician describes the connections between lung cancer and smoking and discusses the urgent need for you to stop smoking *immediately*. What are you feeling as you leave the doctor's office?
- SCENE 5: You are admitted to the hospital for emergency surgery. As you are being prepared for surgery, your lawyer comes in and asks you to describe your last wishes. Tell your lawyer how you wish your property to be disposed of after your death.
- SCENE 6: Your fairy godmother appears to offer you one last chance of continued good health—provided that you make an irreversible commitment to quit smoking immediately. If you promise to quit immediately, she will wave her wand and all the previous events in this ex-

ercise will become only make-believe. What do you say? How do you feel?

The psychologists who devised the role-playing approach suggest that such exercises may serve as an exceptionally valuable tool for the smoker who is trying to quit. What this role-playing does, they believe, is to help break through the psychological defenses that normally prevent smokers from confronting the full and potentially fatal risks they run by continuing to smoke.[28]

Your Last Cigarette

There are several ways to handle this. You may decide that the last cigarette you smoked was your final one. Or you may decide to smoke your last cigarette as part of a ceremony or ritual of your own devising. You may wish to smoke your last cigarette in the company of a special support person. You may wish to invite a few carefully chosen friends to witness your last cigarette. You may, indeed, wish to throw a party to celebrate your last cigarette.

Most successful ex-smokers recommend that you observe *some* kind of ritual in smoking your last cigarette. The ritual can be public or private. San Francisco psychologist David Geisinger suggests that you lock yourself in the bathroom, meditate on the significance of the event, burn your remaining cigarettes in the bathroom basin, then smoke your last cigarette as fast as you possibly can while watching yourself in the bathroom mirror.[29]

Here are some additional steps you may want to take on your quitting day:

- Throw away all your ashtrays.
- Have your teeth cleaned. Ask your dentist to review self-care measures for your teeth and gums.

- Get a professional massage.

- Drink lots of your favorite fruit juices.

- Go for a long walk, either alone or with a key smoking support person.

- Plan nurturing activities for the next 30 days.

- Take a soothing bath or shower.

- Listen to music.

- Drive or ride to work by a new route.

- Have your car cleaned. Wash out the ashtray and fill it with toothpicks.

- Declare your house a nonsmoking area. Buy an attractive NO SMOKING sign and put it near your front door. If you have friends who smoke, establish an outside area for smoking.

- Have the inside of your house—drapes, carpets, furniture—thoroughly cleaned.

Dealing with Withdrawal

Tobacco smokers are in a chronic state of nervous stimulation. Many of the physical symptoms quitters experience are the result of the nervous system returning to normal. These symptoms usually peak by the second or third day and decline thereafter. Symptoms of nicotine withdrawal vary widely from person to person, but may include the following:

- increased appetite, especially for sweet foods;
- increased sputum production;
- cough;
- sweating;

- muscle aches and cramps;
- constipation or diarrhea;
- nausea;
- headache;
- hypersensitivity to physical stimuli;
- sleep disturbances;
- weight gain.

Since smokers are accustomed to obtaining increased concentration and alertness from their cigarettes, some find themselves feeling foggy-headed, unfocused, and forgetful for a short time after quitting. Fortunately, these symptoms also pass their peak by the second or third day, then drop off rapidly.

The best advice for getting through this time is to arrange all possible social, psychological, and environmental support, then to tough it out by whatever means you think best, remembering that in a few days, the great majority of the unpleasant feelings will pass and you will be free of this bothersome—and unhealthy—habit. Other negative psychological symptoms of nicotine withdrawal may include:

- irritability;
- restlessness;
- anxiety;
- increase in aggressive thoughts and behavior;
- depression;
- decreased ability to tolerate stress;
- decreased sexual drive;
- impaired work performance;
- intense cigarette cravings.

Happily, there are many positive psychological symptoms and positive physical effects to counterbalance the negative effects of nicotine withdrawal. They include:

- euphoria at being free of cigarettes;
- decrease in blood pressure;
- decrease in pulse rate;
- better circulation to hands and feet;
- decrease in carbon monoxide blood level;
- more oxygen to the brain and other parts of the body.

In addition, the natural cleansing systems in your lungs begin to operate more effectively. Your sense of smell begins to return. Your food begins to taste better. Your home, office, clothes, hair, and body begin to smell better.

Many successful quitters advise that you will experience a strong urge to have something in your mouth or in your hands. They advise that you lay in a good supply of some of the following:

- E-Z Quit placebo cigarettes (see p. 195);
- sugarless chewing gum;
- carrot sticks, celery, and other crunchy vegetables;
- apples, oranges, bananas, and other fruits;
- cinnamon or licorice sticks;
- fruit juices;
- toothpicks;
- jigsaw or crossword puzzles;
- half a dozen good books.

Other tips:

- Give yourself permission to get through your first week as a nonsmoker in the way that works best for you, no matter how strange or unusual it may seem to others. Treat yourself to whatever you feel like having during this time (other than tobacco and your designated high-risk smoking situations). If you are making efforts to control weight gain during this period, you may also wish to limit your consumption of foods high in fat and sugar.

- Avoid all possible social occasions at which smokers will be present. If you must attend, stay as far as possible from the smokers.

- Review the benefits of quitting several times per day, using the cards described on p. 145.

- Cigarette cravings appear to be mild in the morning. *The period of most intense craving is between noon and 10 P.M., with the peak between 7 and 8 P.M.* Craving is most intense for the first two to three days, then drops off sharply, reaching a substantially reduced level about one week after the last cigarette. Physical and psychological symptoms follow a similar trend.[30]

- Studies show that using nicotine gum can significantly reduce withdrawal symptoms, especially irritability and hunger. Nicotine gum may be especially useful for heavy smokers.[31] (see chapter 8: Nicotine Without Tobacco.)

Why Everything May Seem to Go Wrong After You Quit

Several of the successful ex-smokers we interviewed warned prospective quitters to be open to the possibility that more than the usual number of things may seem to go wrong during the days and weeks after they quit. Although this phenomenon is by no means universal, it was mentioned frequently enough in our interviews to be worth noting here. The "things going wrong" syndrome may be due, in part, to the increased level of irritability, the decreased level of attention, and the sleep disturbances that some ex-smokers experience for the first few days after quitting.

"It's uncanny," one ex-smoker told us. "The leader of my stop-smoking group had told me to expect everything in my life to go wrong at once, but I had no idea to what a remarkable extent this would, in fact, come to pass. A fantastic sequence of improbable events all took place the week after I quit. I got into a series of horrible arguments with my wife, a major customer switched to our main competitor, I received a notice of a tax audit, and the transmission fell out of my car. After awhile, I just had a laugh. It really seemed as though the universe was doing everything it could to give me an excuse to start smoking again."

One smoker cheerfully summed things up as follows: "You should preplan things and protect yourself from outside stresses during the week after you quit as much as you possibly can. But even with the best preplanning, quitting is an extremely unsettling experience. Even under these circumstances it may feel—temporarily at least—as if somebody dropped a bomb on your life."

Maintaining Your Nonsmoking Status

The day you smoke your last cigarette will mark the end of one period of your life and the beginning of another. Because smoking is so closely tied to one's lifestyle, it may be necessary to make changes in many unanticipated areas of your life in order to support your decision to end this unhealthy habit. You may need to modify your daily routines, take up new activities, or drop old ones.

Here are some steps you can take to strengthen your nonsmoking status:

• Set up a regular maintenance ritual one day each week. Sit down with your key support person—or check in by phone. Review your progress so far. Talk about any difficulties you've encountered or anticipate. And re-inforce your desire to remain a nonsmoker. Or you may decide to do this weekly review in your smoking journal.

• Keep a careful lookout for your main cigarette triggers and other obstacles to quitting. Be especially watchful for the following:

—drinking alcohol, especially with others who are smoking;
—frustration or tension at work;
—relaxing after meals;
—periods of depression or boredom;
—self-pity;
—switching to other forms of tobacco;
—social pressure to smoke;
—offering to buy or hold cigarettes for a smoking friend.

• Make a special effort to make and extend friendships with nonsmokers and ex-smokers.

• Make a bet or other pact with a close friend or relative, specifying a reward or celebration that will mark your successful completion of six months or a full year without cigarettes.

• Make a public announcement of your intention to quit to a club, religious or other group to which you feel a close bond or to individuals you respect.

• Ask others not to smoke in your house or car.

Dealing with Slips

If you *do* experience a slip, don't fall victim to the so-called abstinence violation effect. In this all-too-common pattern of self-defeatist thinking, a single slip triggers a period of intense self-castigation, depression, and negativity (I'm no good, I have no willpower, I wasn't really cured anyway, etc.). This, in turn, leads to a decreased sense of control, a drop in self-esteem, and further slips, until the person abandons all efforts to quit.[32].

A slip is a two-step process—a smoking risk situation plus an inadequate coping response. A slip or two on the way to eventual success does not make you a failure. The only real failure would be giving up your efforts to quit. If you do find yourself slipping, simply catch yourself and take control again.[33] Accept the fact that you have slipped, let it go, and allow yourself to return to your nonsmoking state without recriminations or self-blame. This "no-fault" approach will increase your chances of ultimate success. Many people who eventually succeed experience dozens of such slips on the way to their goal.

Very few slips (only 2 to 9 percent) occur because of physical withdrawal symptoms. Most occur when you are anxious, angry, frustrated, or depressed—especially if, at such times, you are offered a cigarette (or alcohol first and a cigarette later) by a well-meaning friend.

Here are some good ways to avoid slips:[34]

- Do your best to stay away from high-risk situations, such as going to a bar where others are smoking and drinking.

- Recognize a relapse crisis when you see one. Review your nonsmoking coping strategies, choose the best one, and put it into action.

- Be on the lookout for "apparently irrelevant de-

cisions'' to hold a burning cigarette for a friend
or to buy cigarettes for a friend who still smokes.
Such decisions can lead to slips. Resolve to have
nothing whatsoever to do with cigarettes for the
first few months after you quit.

The Rewards of Quitting

The benefits of quitting begin immediately. The carbon
monoxide level in your blood returns to normal within
12 hours. Your heart rate slows and your skin tempera-
ture increases. Cardiac function, peripheral circulation,
and fine motor coordination all improve within the first
day.[35]

"The day you quit painting your tracheobronchial tree
with chemicals that cause cancer is the day you begin
recovery,'' says pathologist Oscar Auerbach, a senior
medical investigator at the Veterans Administration Medical Center in East Orange, N.J. Auerbach's research has
helped document the reversibility of damage produced
by smoking. And Dr. William P. Castelli, medical director of the Framingham heart study, says that the improvement in a smoker's heart begins within a few days.
Ex-smokers' hearts can return to a nearly normal condition within a year after quitting.

The first thing quitters notice is that they can breathe
again, says Dr. William G. Cahan, Professor Emeritus at
Cornell University School of Medicine. Quitters usually
notice the difference within two or three weeks, Dr. Cahan says. Other benefits during the first few weeks include the return of your lost senses of taste and smell.
Your breath will smell better. Other respiratory symptoms will gradually disappear. Your immune system will
show improved functioning levels within three months.[36]

Your stamina and vigor continue to improve over the

next two to three months. Headaches and stomachaches caused by smoking will disappear. You will continue to notice increased health and improved well being for six to eight months.

You will experience a 90 percent drop in your risk of heart disease within the first year, a truly massive decrease. If you are able to make changes in your eating habits and exercise and stress levels during this time, the possible risk reduction can be even greater.[37] Within ten to fifteen years, your risk of lung cancer will be roughly the same as if you had never smoked.[38] In the long run, ex-smokers will also reduce their risk of all other smoking-related diseases described in chapter 3.

Other Encouraging Factors

As the facts above demonstrate, virtually all of the negative health effects of smoking are reversible. Quitting *is* possible. Over a million Americans have done it every year for the past twenty years. You can too.

We'd like to end this chapter by quoting two stanzas from "It Couldn't Be Done," a poem by Edgar A. Guest that one successful ex-smoker sent us.

"This little ditty convinced me to quit," she wrote. "It really was a big help—along with regular exercise, nicotine gum, and some very loving and supportive friends—in getting through the tough days after I *did* quit.

"I typed it out, changing the 'he' to 'she,' made a number of copies, and kept them on my refrigerator door, my bathroom mirror, and in my purse. I hope you can include it in your book. I think others might find it equally useful."

Somebody said that it couldn't be done
But he with a chuckle replied
That maybe it couldn't, but he would be one
Who wouldn't say so till he'd tried.

So he buckled right in with the trace of a grin
On his face. If he worried, he hid it.
He started to sing as he tackled the thing
That couldn't be done. And he did it.

Suggested Activities for Each of the
Ten Stages of Quitting

Stage One: You have identified yourself as a health-concerned smoker.

· Pay attention to the role smoking plays in your life.
· Seek out opportunities to talk about smoking with others.
· Observe the ways nonsmokers respond to situations to which you respond by smoking.
· Observe other smokers carefully, paying special attention to the negative aspects of the habit.
· Smoke in front of a mirror, watching yourself closely from the first puff to the last. What exactly is it that goes on when you smoke a cigarette?

Stage Two: You have decided that you will seek information about healthier alternatives.

· Read through *The No-Nag, No-Guilt, Do-It-Your-Own-Way Guide to Quitting Smoking*, marking sections that seem especially useful to you and making notes in the blank pages at the back or in a separate notebook.
· Seek out friends who have recently quit smoking. Ask them to describe how they did it.
· Choose one risk-reduction step from chapters 5, 6, or 7 and put it into practice.
· Tell one close friend that you are exploring healthier alternatives to smoking.
· When you feel an urge for a cigarette, wait one minute before lighting up. Experience the urge fully and think of other ways you might respond to it.
· Begin to reward yourself for becoming more aware of your smoking patterns and for learning about more healthful alternatives.

Stage Three: You have decided to take some steps to modify your smoking risk (switching brands, cutting down, getting more exercise, taking vitamins, etc.).

- Begin keeping a smoking journal in which you write down your thoughts about smoking.
- Become aware of times when you find yourself smoking more or less than usual.
- Begin collecting and trying new stress reduction techniques.
- Adopt a healthful new activity that is incompatible with smoking (swimming, going to concerts, joining a singing group).
- Switch to a lower tar brand. Be careful not to smoke more heavily as compensation for reduced nicotine intake.
- Reward yourself for each smoking reduction or risk modification.

Stage Four: You decide that you will quit at an unspecified date in the near future.

- Reward yourself for making a commitment to quit.
- Begin keeping track of the number of cigarettes you smoke each day.
- Stop buying cartons. Buy only one pack at a time.
- Identify your top cigarette triggers.
- Buy a new toothbrush or toothpaste and begin brushing your teeth several times per day.
- List the reasons you'd like to quit.
- Begin switching brands every week. Each new brand should be lower in tar than the last. Again, be careful not to increase your smoking to make up for lower nicotine levels.
- Postpone every third cigarette.
- Begin talking with your closest friends and family members about your intention to quit. Suggest ways they could help in your effort to quit.

Stage Five: Set a quitting date and make a firm commitment to quit on that date.

- Give yourself a big reward for setting your quitting date.
- Sign a stop-smoking contract. See chapter 10 for sample contracts.
- Ask to be seated in the nonsmoking sections of restaurants and airplanes.

- Prepare at least three alternative responses for each of your top ten cigarette triggers.
- Set up a health bank. See chapter 10 for details.
- Increase your level of daily activity.
- Begin switching brands with every pack.
- Postpone every other cigarette.
- Follow the guidelines for controlled smoking offered in chapter 5.
- Begin cutting back on alcoholic beverages.
- Begin adopting the alternative responses you have selected when confronted by your cigarette triggers.

Stage Six: You smoke your last cigarette and go without smoking for 24 hours.

- Pamper yourself as much as possible. Treat yourself as someone special.
- Use your key social support people.
- Work on defusing your cigarette triggers.
- Schedule healthy activities (long walks, bike rides, a ball game, fishing, dancing, browsing in your favorite shops, lunch in the nonsmoking section of a special restaurant).
- Have your teeth cleaned.
- Send your favorite articles of clothing to the cleaners.
- Discard all your ashtrays.
- If you have chosen to do so, begin using nicotine gum or another tobaccoless nicotine source (see chapter 8 for details).
- Get a friend to help you practice saying no when offered a cigarette.

Stage Seven: You complete your first week as a nonsmoker.

- Continue working on defusing your cigarette triggers.
- Find additional ways to use your key social support people.
- Indulge yourself in daily rewards, treats, and pleasant activities.
- Stay away from places where people are likely to be smoking.
- Schedule massages, hot baths, exercise, etc.
- Notice how much better your food tastes.
- Continue to notice and celebrate improvements in your health.

Stage Eight: You complete your first month as a non-smoker.

- If you haven't already done so, begin a regular exercise program.
- Each week add one new stress-reduction technique to your activities.
- Celebrate your success with your key support people. Tell them about the positive feelings and health improvements you're experiencing.
- Continue to avoid places where people will be drinking and smoking.

Stage Nine: You complete your first three months as a nonsmoker.

- Continue to gently increase your exercise level.
- Treat yourself to a relaxing weekend getaway.
- Let your friends who smoke know that if they'd be interested in discussing cutting down or quitting, you'd be happy to talk with them.
- Continue to notice and celebrate improvements in your health.
- (At five to six months) If you have been using nicotine gum or some other nicotine replacement, begin cutting back.

Stage Ten: You complete your first year as a nonsmoker.

- Offer to be the principal support person for a friend who wants to quit.
- Call your local American Cancer Society chapter and volunteer to help others quit.
- Throw a party to celebrate your first year as a nonsmoker.
- If you have not already done so, taper off and then stop using your nicotine substitute. You may wish to keep a small supply on hand "in case of emergency."

Becoming a Permanent Nonsmoker

9

Nicotine Without Tobacco: Using Nicorette Brand Nicotine Gum

If you regularly inhale more than ten cigarettes per day, you're an addicted smoker. But it's *nicotine* you're addicted to, not tobacco.

Nicotine is the principal psychoactive substance in tobacco smoke, but nicotine itself, in the doses most smokers receive, appears to produce little or no harm in the otherwise healthy smoker. Studies to date suggest that it is the *tar, carbon monoxide, and other toxic gases* which are responsible for the great majority of tobacco-related disease. Pharmacologist Neal L. Benowitz of San Francisco General Hospital, one of the scientific editors of the most recent Surgeon General's Report, sums it up this way: "Nicotine *could* play a role in the pathogenesis of many smoking-related diseases, although at present there is no conclusive evidence that it contributes to *any*."[1]

Well guess what? Modern science has come to the smoker's rescue. There *is* a way to get your accustomed dose of nicotine without touching another cigarette.

There *is* a way to give up cigarettes without giving up all the psychological benefits of nicotine or going through the kind of withdrawal you'd experience if you quit "cold turkey."

The development of nontobacco sources of nicotine is the most hopeful and promising new tool for health-concerned smokers since the filter-tip.[2] As we go to press, the prescription drug Nicorette, a sustained-release, nicotine-containing oral resin, is the only available product which employs this approach. Possible future products, still in the research stage, are described below.

Nicorette has produced considerable excitement among smoking researchers. The dean of smoking research, British psychiatrist M.A.H. Russell, writing with his colleague M.J. Jarvis, has stated: "In our view, [Nicorette] is the most significant single advance achieved so far in the whole field of smoking cessation." Researcher Nina Schneider of UCLA calls it "the first viable aid to smoking cessation."[3]

Nicorette provides a welcome "third way" for health-concerned smokers. Before Nicorette, smokers had only two choices: you could smoke or you could quit cold turkey. Now there are *three* alternatives: you can smoke; you can quite cold turkey; or you can switch from tobacco to Nicorette, and then gradually withdraw from the Nicorette.

Quitting Without Withdrawal

By obtaining a prescription form Nicorette, you can now break the quitting process down into two manageable stages: In stage one, you will smoke your last cigarette and will begin getting your nicotine from Nicorette. In stage two, you will gradually taper down and discontinue the Nicorette, which is substantially less addictive than cigarettes. By going through a prolonged period in which you are tobacco-free but can still have a dose of nicotine whenever you wish, you can take the time to focus on overcoming the behavioral and psychological components of the smoking habit without having to go through nicotine withdrawal at the same time. You can then wean yourself from the Nicorette at a later date, when you no longer experience an overpowering urge to smoke.[4]

About Nicorette

You may have heard Nicorette referred to as "nicotine chewing gum." We suggest that you should *not* think of Nicorette as a chewing gum. It is, technically speaking, an "oral resin containing a transmucosal sustained-release medication." This is a new kind of drug delivery system. It *looks* like gum, but you don't *chew* it like gum. *Chewing Nicorette like gum makes it much less effective and increases the risk of side effects.*

To use Nicorette effectively there are several important things you must know:

• Nicotine is released from the Nicorette when a freshly-exposed surface comes in contact with saliva. Thus, while you will need to chew a new piece of Nicorette a few times when you first put it in your mouth, you need only give it an occasional gentle bite—to expose a fresh surface—thereafter.

• When you first put a new piece of Nicorette in your mouth, you should chew it just enough to soften the medication and trigger the release of the nicotine. This usually requires chewing about ten to twelve times. As soon as you begin to feel a spicy taste or "tingling" in your mouth, *stop chewing* and "park" the Nicorette in your cheek.

• In order to be effective, the nicotine from the Nicorette must be absorbed through the membrane on the inside of your cheek. The Nicorette acts like an internal "skin patch," providing a slow release of nicotine which is absorbed through your cheek and into your blood. Keep the Nicorette in your cheek until the "tingling" or spicy taste goes away.

• When the tingling has completely disappeared, bite the Nicorette gently once or twice to restart the release of nicotine. Vigorous chewing is not necessary. Stop when you feel the tingle. Again, park the Nicorette in your cheek.

• Repeat this process until you no longer feel the tingle when you bite or chew the Nicorette. Each piece lasts for approximately 30 minutes, although this varies from person to person.

• Any nicotine which is swallowed with saliva or washed down while eating or drinking will not be effective. If a substantial amount of nicotine is swallowed, it may cause such side-effects as heartburn, upset stomach, or hiccups. Thus you should not eat or drink while you have Nicorette in your mouth.

Nicorette: What's In It?

Nicorette is manufactured by the Swedish drug company A.B. Leo, which first developed it. It is distributed in the United States and Canada by Lakeside Pharmaceuticals, a division of Merrell Dow Pharmaceuticals of Cincinnati. The gum is also in widespread use in Canada, Great Britain, Switzerland, Sweden, and roughly forty other countries. In the United States, the gum is sold in tablets containing 2mg. of nicotine and is available only by prescription.

Nicorette contains an ordinary chewing-gum base, but in addition contains nicotine bound to an ion-exchange resin. As the result of chewing and contact with saliva, molecules of nicotine are gradually dislodged from the resin. The nicotine is then absorbed into the bloodstream through the membranes that line of the inside of the mouth. The gum also contains a buffer which insures that the nicotine will be absorbed at a steady rate.

Nicorette: How Effective?

In a study published in 1982 in the *British Medical Journal*, researchers subjected Nicorette to a controlled, double-blind study. Half of their subjects received 2mg. doses. The other half received a nicotine flavored, but pharmacologically inactive gum made up into identical tablets. Neither the researchers who met with the subjects nor the subjects themselves knew which subjects were receiving which type of gum. Both groups were also invited to attend small group meetings once a week for six weeks.

A year later the researchers evaluated the smoking status of all subjects. They found that more than twice as many of those who had received the nicotine gum succeeded in quitting: 47% of those who had received Nicorette had become long-term nonsmokers, compared to 21% of those who had received the inactive form of the gum. In addition, those who had received Nicorette reported significantly fewer withdrawal symptoms during the first six weeks after quitting.[6]

Fewer Withdrawal Symptoms

Other researchers have noted similar results. Using Nicorette seems to roughly double a smoker's chances of successful long-term quitting. In addition, the gum significantly decreases the severity of such withdrawal symptoms as irritability, anger, frustration, restlessness, impatience, sleepiness, and food cravings. A number of studies also suggest that the gum can significantly reduce, though it does not completely eliminate, the craving for cigarettes.[7]

Nicorette appears to be particularly effective in decreasing withdrawal symptoms during the afternoon and evening hours. This makes the gum especially useful, since withdrawal symptoms characteristically become more intense during the later part of the day.

No Panacea

If you want to quit smoking. Nicorette can be a powerful aid. But this medication is an *aid* to quitting, not a cure. In spite of the high enthusiasm shown by researchers and the encouraging success rates among prospective quitters who used Nicorette, you must understand that the gum will not "do it for you." As Russell and Jarvis write, "the gum is at best a partial substitute for cigarettes and does not provide as much positive satisfaction. It follows that it is a treatment aid rather than a complete treatment. Smokers who approach it naively, hoping, as many do, that it will somehow magically stop their smoking without the need for any effort on their part, are inevitably disappointed any may wrongly conclude that the gum has nothing at all to offer.[8]

One ex-smoker who used nicotine gum as an aid in quitting put it this way: "Smokers need to know right up front that chewing the gum is *not* the same as having a cigarette. When you light up, you get that nice feeling of satisfaction right away. With the gum it takes longer, and its less intense. Using Nicorette doesn't exactly make you stop *wanting* a cigarette. But it makes it a whole lot more bearable not to *have* one.''

Nicorette does *not* eliminate the need for alternative healthful activities, new thinking patterns, and intense social and psychological support for the six to twelve months after quitting. Here are some of the kinds of support that seems to be most important:

• Recording and reviewing your pattern of Nicorette use.

• Learning and using new stress management skills.

• Getting together with a key support person to discuss potential problems and brainstorm possible solutions.

• Avoiding high-risk relapse situations.

• Reinforcing your commitment to continue Nicorette use. (Smokers who use Nicorette for less than four months are more likely to relapse.)

• Beginning again immediately if slips do occur.

Are You a Candidate for Nicorette?

The Swedish smoking researcher Karl-Olov Fagerstrom has developed a self-scoring quiz to help smokers determine their present dependence on nicotine.[9] Most researchers would agree that the more addicted a smoker is, the more the nicotine gum should help.

Questions	Answers	Points	Score
1. How soon after you wake do you smoke your first cigarette?	Within 30 minutes	1	_____
	After 30 minutes	0	_____
2. Do you find it difficult to refrain from smoking in places where it is forbidden?	Yes	1	_____
	No	0	_____

3. Which cigarette would you hate to give up most?	The first one in the morning	1	____
	Any other	0	____
4. How many cigarettes a day do you smoke?	15 or less	0	____
	16–25	1	____
	26 or more	2	____
5. Do you smoke more frequently during the early morning than during the rest of the day?	Yes	1	____
	No	0	____
6. Do you smoke if you are so ill that you are in bed most of the day?	Yes	1	____
	No	0	____
7. What is the nicotine level of your usual brand of cigarettes?	0.9 mg or less	0	____
	1.0–1.2 mg	1	____
	1.3 mg or more	2	____
8. Do you inhale?	Never	0	____
	Sometimes	1	____
	Always	2	____
		Total:	____

Scoring:	0–5	Low dependence level
	6–7	Medium dependence level
	7–11	High dependence level

How to Get a Prescription for Nicotine Gum

Any licensed physician or dentist can write a prescription for Nicorette. You may already have a doctor or dentist you like and trust. If not, you may wish to find a physician or dentist who takes special interest in smoking cessation and who is knowledgeable and experienced about the use of nicotine gum.

One good way to find such a doctor is to call your local

chapter of the American Lung Association, the American Cancer Society, or the American Heart Association. Or call one of the agencies listed under ''Smoker's Information and Treatment Centers'' in your local yellow pages. Or ask your local pharmacist to recommend a doctor or dentist.

Nicotine gum is currently sold without prescription in Switzerland. Some industry insiders speculate that the gum's U.S. distributor, Lakeside Pharmaceuticals, may eventually apply for OTC status for the product.[10]

Guidelines for Using Nicotine Gum

Some smokers find the taste of Nicorette a bit disagreeable the first few times. This may be because you are chewing the Nicorette like gum rather than as directed. But don't give up. Stay with it. As the days go by and you become more adept at using Nicorette, it will become less bothersome and more satisfying. Study the guidelines below and the instructions that come with your prescription *thoroughly*. Above all, remember that using Nicorette will not *make* you stop smoking. For this medication to be effective, it must be used *after* you quit.

How to Use Nicorette[11]

0–4 months	• Chew Nicorette whenever you wish, but do not exceed 30 pieces per day. (Moderate smokers usually experience best results if they chew 8 to 20 pieces per day. Heavy smokers may find they need to chew 20 to 30 pieces per day.)
4–6 months	• Gradually begin to taper down on the gum.

| 6–12 months | • Taper down to 1 or 2 pieces per day. When you feel ready, discontinue the gum. But carry a few pieces with you at all times as a "security blanket"—and chew it if you experience a strong urge to smoke. |
| 1 year & beyond | • Discontinue Nicorette except for emergencies. Keep a few pieces in a convenient place so you can use it if you experience intense cravings. |

Remember: Nicorette is not ordinary chewing gum. It is a sophisticated drug delivery device. The only time you will need to chew Nicorette is when you first put a fresh piece into your mouth. (It usually takes about 12 to 15 chews before you taste the nicotine, but this varies from person to person.) After that, you will only need to bite it when the flavor goes away in order to expose a fresh surface. Most of the time you have Nicorette in your mouth it should be "parked" in your cheek.

Warnings and Precautions

• If you chew Nicorette like regular chewing gum, you may experience unpleasant side effects similar to those people get when they smoke a cigarette for the first time. Symptoms of too much nicotine may include:

  —Dizziness or lightheadedness.
  —Nausea and vomiting.
  —Irritation of the mouth and throat.
  —Hiccups.

• Other side effects sometimes seen, especially within the first few days—include:

  —Aching jaw muscles from chewing the gum for long periods.

—Soreness or ulceration of the mouth.

—Headaches.

—Loud or rapid beating of the heart.

—Excessive salivation.

—Belching as the result of swallowing air while chewing the gum.

• Report any other bothersome symptoms to the physician or dentist who prescribed the gum.

• Women should take precautions to avoid pregnancy while using the nicotine gum. If you suspect you *have* become pregnant, discontinue use immediately and consult your physician or dentist.

• Nicorette gum is stickier than some other kinds of gum and may stick to or damage dental work or pull out fillings. If you have dentures, bridges, or braces, you may wish to obtain your prescription from your dentist so that you can ask for special advice.

• Do not swallow the gum. Adverse effects are unlikely, but if you do swallow a piece and begin to experience adverse effects, contact a physician or your local poison control center at once. Overdose could occur if many pieces are chewed or swallowed in a short period of time.

• Keep Nicorette away from children. If a child accidentally chews or swallows a piece of Nicorette, contact a physician or your local poison control center immediately.

Side Effects of Nicorette[12]

Symptom	% Nicorette Users Reporting	% Placebo Users Reporting
Felt sick	38	20
Been sick	4	0
Dizziness	21	18
Sore throat	40	39
Headache	30	39
Sore mouth	60	52
Felt faint	11	7
Hiccups	30	5
Indigestion	51	27
Tiredness from chewing	53	59
Mouth ulcers	2	2
Dependence on Nicorette	7	0

Nicotine Gum—What Does It Cost?

If you get your prescription from a discount pharmacy, Nicorette will probably cost just a bit more than you're now spending for cigarettes. As we go to press, Austin, Texas, prices for a 96-piece box of Nicorette range from a high of $32.30 at our neighborhood pharmacy to a low of $18.45 at our local Wal-Mart. That works out between 19 and 34 cents per piece. Thus the pack-a-day smoker who quit and began chewing twelve pieces of gum a day would switch from a daily cigarette bill of $1.50 to a daily Nicorette bill of $2.25.

How Long Should You Chew the Gum?

Researcher M.A.H. Russell, who probably knows as much about Nicorette as anyone in the world, suggests you continue chewing the gum for at least four months, then decide for yourself when to stop using it. Smokers who do so have a better chance of quitting for good. About seven percent of ex-smokers who use Nicorette to quit smoking are still chewing the gum one year after their last cigarette. Russell believes that this should not be considered a serious problem, since the gum is so much safer than cigarettes. However, he does advise those who are still using Nicorette twelve months after their last cigarette to discontinue the gum as soon as they can.[13]

Recent studies at the University of Minnesota suggest that it is best to discontinue Nicorette gradually, not abruptly. It the gum is stopped suddenly, the user may develop withdrawal symptoms similar to those experienced by smokers who quit "cold turkey"—including irritability, anxiety, restlessness, impatience, and difficulty concentrating. When you are ready to discontinue the gum, you should taper down gradually before stopping altogether.[14]

Other Nontobacco Sources of Nicotine

Researchers are currently studying several other ways of providing ex-smokers with nicotine:

The Favor Inhaler—The Favor brand "smokeless cigarette" is a cigarette-shaped plastic cylinder that contains no tobacco. A small perforated chamber within the "cigarette" is packed with an inert fibrous material saturated with a nicotine solution.

This device was commercially available in some states for eighteen months in 1986 and 1987, but it was taken off the market by the FDA because the manufacturers had not filed a new drug application. It is not currently available. According to the manufacturer, a smoker who puffs on a Favor receives a dose of vaporized nicotine roughly equivalent to that delivered by a low-tar cigarette. But as the Favor is not lit and contains no tobacco, it gives off no tar or carbon monoxide. Each Favor produces four to six times as many pharmacologically active puffs as a regular cigarette. Since Favors are not lit, a smoker can continue using a single Favor until the nicotine in the chamber is exhausted. Thereafter the Favor becomes an inert placebo cigarette which can still be puffed and handled. An article by M.A.H. Russell in the *Journal of the American Medical Association* concluded that with intense puffing, Favor is capable of producing a blood nicotine level comparable to that achieved by smokers.[15] The rights to Favor were recently acquired by the A.B. Leo, the Swedish drug company that developed Nicorette. Research on this device is currently being carried out at Advanced Tobacco Products, Inc., of San Antonio, Texas. A company spokesman said that the company plans to re-introduce an improved version at a later date.[16]

Nicotine Skin Patch

Studies by Jed E. Rose and colleagues at UCLA have found that a skin patch containing nicotine can decrease nicotine craving. They believe that transdermal nicotine delivered by a skin patch might ease the cigarette craving smokers experience after they quit. Advantages of this approach include a relative lack of adverse side effects and the ability of a skin patch to provide constant delivery over a 24-hour period. Nicotine skin patches are cur-

rently undergoing clinical testing in Dr. Rose's laboratory
at UCLA. Several drug companies—Lakeside, A.B. Leo,
and Ciba-Geigy—are also working to develop a nicotine
skin patch. If current tests are successful, the nicotine
skin patch may become available in the near future.[18]

Aerosol Sprays

Dr. Rose of UCLA is also currently doing research on a
variety of aerosol sprays which a smoker can inhale to
simulate the sensations derived from smoking. Some of
the sprays being tested contain a nicotine-containing con-
densate from real cigarette smoke. Others contain citric
acid. The sprays are designed to simulate the taste and
flavor of smoking while reducing or eliminating the toxic
substances to which the smoker is exposed. There are
presently no plans to make these sprays commercially
available.[19]

Nasal Nicotine Solution

When English smoking researcher M.A.H. Russell and
colleagues studied English snuff users—who sniff a finely
powdered form of tobacco through their noses—they
found that they were able to obtain nicotine blood levels
considerably higher than those found in users of nicotine
gum. They proceeded to develop a nasal nicotine solution. Recent studies indicate that this nontobacco substance can also produce nicotine blood levels comparable
to those achieved by smokers.

"It's rather like taking nose drops," Russell explains.
"You put the device into your nose, give a squeeze, and
it delivers a single dose. If you want a bigger dose, you

can squeeze one into each nostril. It's a bit irritating at first, but then people get used to it and grow to like it.''

According to preliminary studies, the nasal nicotine solution is absorbed more quickly and users are able to attain higher nicotine blood levels than with the gum. However, some smokers reported that they were embarrassed to use the nasal nicotine solution while in the company of others. Russell and his co-workers are currently working with the Swedish pharmaceutical company A.B. Leo, the original developers of the nicotine gum, to refine, test, and market the product.[20]

10
Tools and Tips to Help You Quit

There are dozens of products and devices that purport to help smokers quit. Here's our pick of the very best.

E-Z Quit

E-Z Quit consists of a simulated tortoise shell cigarette holder and a plastic "cigarette" containing a pepermint-menthol flavor capsule. Feel like a cigarette? Puff away on an E-Z Quit instead. No smoke, no ashes, no nicotine, and—best of all—*no* damaging health effects. The E-Z Quit can be used either while cutting down or after quitting.

Because there's no smoke, you can even puff away in no-smoking areas. The device itself lasts indefinitely, although the mint flavor disappears after three to four weeks. A 90 day supply of flavor capsules is included. Additional flavor capsules are available.

The smokers in our survey gave the E-Z Quit the highest rating of any non-prescription quit-smoking aid. In fact, the only problem with the E-Z Quit seems to be that they are *so* popular that your friends who smoke may try to "borrow" yours. Even many nonsmokers—my dear wife included—like to puff on these gadgets. Of the several types of "placebo cigarettes" currently on the market, this is far and away the best.

You can order the E-Z Quit for $12.95 postpaid from the Center for Self-Care Studies, 3805 Stevenson Ave., Austin TX 78703, (512) 458–9333.

LifeSign Quit-Smoking Computer

For the technologically minded smoker who wants to quit, the LifeSign may be the answer. This tiny computer, the size of a fat credit card, is programmed to help you taper down gradually before quitting. Several weeks before your chosen quitting day, you press a button to activate the mechanism, then carry the LifeSign with you at all times. For the first week, you press the "smoke" button on the device each time you light a cigarette. Beginning on the first day of the second week, you smoke only when the computer tells you it's time to do so—the computer beeps each time a cigarette is allowed.

It starts you out at your normal smoking rate. The intervals between cigarettes gets longer and longer over a period of two to four weeks immediately before your chosen quitting day. On your quit day and thereafter, the device flashes a "no smoking" symbol.

The LifeSign sells for approximately $80. For more information, write or call Health Innovations, 13873 Park Center Road, Suite 336, Herndon VA 22071, (800) 543-3744, (703) 478-2824.

Lung Check

This home sputum test is designed to serve as an early warning system for smokers by identifying tissue damage at a time when quitting smoking can still reverse the progression of the disease. In addition to screening for lung cancer, the test looks for signs of six other biological responses to cigarette smoke.

The Lung Check is designed to be repeated at regular intervals. Test results are given in a graphic format which allows the smoker to evaluate positive or negative trends in lung function. The test can thus be used by smokers to determine the extent of existing damage or by recent quitters to document improvemant in lung function.

The Lung Check is being marketed primarily to physicians although the company will also provide the test directly to interested individuals. Those who order the test will receive a stamped, mail-in sputum container, a brochure on smoking and your lungs, and instructions for collecting a sputum sample. The user collects three morning sputum samples and mails them back to the lab. The results arrive by mail.

You just include the name and phone number of your primary physician with your order. The lab will phone your physician if the results suggest that further testing may be needed.

The test costs approximately $46. Health insurance, Medicare, and Medicaid will pay for the test if it is ordered by a physician.

For more information on the test, write or call: CytoSciences, Lung Check Division, 1601 Saratoga Sunnyvale Rd., Cupertino CA 95014, (800) 433-8278, (408) 996-0600.

Residential Treatment Centers for Smokers

We've received many questions from readers asking about residential centers where smokers might go to quit smoking in a supportive, sympathetic, structured environment. We've heard of only a few centers and have been unable to locate a directory of residential smoking programs. Thus we've decided to compile such a directory ourselves. We'd like to ask your help.

If you know of a residential treatment center providing programs for smokers who wish to quit, please let us know. If you're been through such a program, please share your experiences with us. If you are associated with such a center, please send us information on your program—including length, fees, program description, contact person, address, phone number, and other relevant details. If you know of materials, studies, guidelines, or advice that should be included in such a directory, please send it along. To obtain a copy of the directory, please send $2.00 to: Residential Smoking Program Directory, Center for Self-Care Studies, 3805 Stevenson Ave., Austin TX 78703, (512) 458-9333.

Health Bank

This method provides financial rewards for positive steps taken toward quitting. As part of your commitment to quit, you pledge to put aside a specified sum each week. This money can be kept in a special envelope or bank account or you can ask a friend to keep it for you. You receive the money when you have gone without smoking for 100 days (or any other length of time you prefer). You may wish to ask some of your support people to contribute to your health bank.

A group of New Jersey smokers recently invented an interesting variation of the health bank idea. Six coworkers at Princeton's Center for Health Affairs quit smoking the same day. Each put $100 into a kitty held by a nonsmoking colleague. Four months after their quitting date, the money will be divided equally among those members who have remained nonsmokers.

Lung Ashtray

This device consists of two transparent plastic lungs mounted over an ashtray. As smoke from a cigarette rises, it passes through one lung but not the other. The buildup of tar in the affected lung, in contrast to the clean lung, graphically illustrates what happens in the lungs of a smoker. The lung ashtray sells for approximately $12. Write to HealthEdCo, P.O. Box 21207, Waco, Texas 76702, or call (800) 433-2677.

Mechanical Smoker

This inexpensive teaching device does a remarkable job of showing you exactly what smoking does to your lungs. Insert a lighted cigarette into its cardbord "mouth," pump its "body" (a small plastic air pump), and it will "smoke" the cigarette, depositing the resulting tar in a transparent plastic "mini lung." The device comes with 100 mini-lungs and a 20-page lesson guide (additional mini-lungs are available). It too is offered by HealthEdCo (address above), and sells for approximately $20.

The Rubber Band Method

A recent American Cancer Society contest to come up with new ideas on how to break the smoking habit was won by Mrs. Janet MacAinsh of Howell, Michigan, who said that she had broken her twenty-six-year pack-a-day habit with the help of a rubber band. She kept the rubber band on her wrist and snapped it against her skin whenever she felt the urge to light up. Be sure the rubber band is loose enough that it doesn't block blood flow or leave a mark on the skin when it is removed. According to Edward Lichtenstein of the University of Oregon, preliminary research suggests that this approach really does help people quit.[1]

Clonidine

A study conducted by Alexander Glassman and his colleagues at Columbia University found that the drug clonidine (marketed under the brand name Catapres) significantly reduced withdrawal symptoms and nicotine cravings among recent quitters. Clonidine is frequently prescribed for high blood pressure.

This study is worth describing in some detail: Fifteen heavy smokers (more than 30 cigarettes per day) were asked not to smoke after going to bed the night before they were due to report to the research laboratory. When they reported to the lab the next morning, they were given either clonidine (0.2 mg. in two divided doses 90 minutes apart) or a placebo. Neither the subjects nor the researchers knew which subjects were getting clonidine.

The subjects were then asked to rate themselves once an hour for their levels of tension, anxiety, irritability, craving for cigarettes, restlessness, impaired concentration, sadness, drowsiness, and dizziness. At the end of the day they were asked to rate the degree to which the treatment they received helped them do without cigarettes. Each smoker received clonidine on one occasion and the placebo on a different day. The subjects' average ratings on the nine scales were as follows:

Scale 1–10	Clonidine	Placebo
Anxiety	1.46	2.94
Irritability	2.20	3.91
Craving	3.24	6.03
Restlessness	1.60	3.09
Impaired concentration	2.17	2.27
Sadness	0.83	0.72
Tension	1.51	3.12
Drowsiness	5.06	1.13
Dizziness	2.58	1.15
"How much did the treatment help?"	7.3	2.8

The nicotine-deprived smokers who received clonidine felt only about 40 percent of the urge to smoke as those who received the placebo; 27 percent of the subjects receiving clonidine said they felt *no urge to smoke at all*. None of the subjects receiving the placebo reported this finding. Dizziness and drowsiness was much more common among the subjects who received clonidine. These are common side effects of the drug.

Clonidine seems to have an even more powerful effect in reducing cigarette cravings later in the day. And since cigarette cravings in recent quitters tend to become stronger as the day goes on, the researchers note that this may make clonidine a major cessation aid. Clonidine has its maximum urge-suppression effect exactly at the time when tobacco-deprived smokers need it the most.

The researchers warn, however, that their results do

not imply clonidine is a "cure" for smoking. Some hypertensive patients taking clonidine do continue to smoke. "However," they wrote, "any drug that could enable heavy smokers to abstain quickly and relatively asymptomatically is potentially clinically useful."[2]

As we go to press, smoking cessation has not been listed as an approved use for clonidine. However, it has been widely used by some physicians in helping people withdraw from a number of addictive substances—including cigarettes.

If you *are* receiving medical treatment for hypertension, ask your doctor if it would be appropriate for you to switch to clonidine. Some physicians may be willing to prescribe clonidine for prospective quitters even if they do not have hypertension—particularly those with serious smoking-related illnesses (such as emphysema) who have been unable to quit by other means.

The patent on clonidine is due to expire about the time this book is published, so this drug may soon be available generically and under brand names other than Catapres.[3]

Stop-Smoking Groups

Action on Smoking and Health (ASH)
2013 H Street, NW
Washington, DC 20006
(202) 659–4310

Action on Smoking and Health is the leading antismoking consumer group in the United States. The organization provides support for antismoking activists and seeks to promote legal changes that will protect the nonsmoker's right to breathe fresh air. ASH also sells buttons and bumperstrips with antismoking messages and a variety of NO SMOKING signs. The ASH newsletter is one of the best available sources of current news on smoking and health and antismoking activism. A yearly subscription costs $5.00.

American Lung Association
1740 Broadway
New York, NY 10019
(212) 315–8700

The American Lung Association sponsors stop-smoking groups in most cities. It also publishes an excellent guide to quitting, *Freedom From Smoking for You and Your Family*. This book guides readers through a step-by-step 20-day program that leads to quitting and provides guidelines for remaining a nonsmoker. The book is available from your local chapter of the American Lung Association (consult your telephone directory for the address and phone number) or from their national headquarters at the address above.

American Cancer Society
4 West 35th Street
New York, NY 10001
(212) 736–3030

Local affiliates of the American Cancer Society sponsor a four-session stop-smoking program called Fresh-Start. Sessions last one hour each and extend over a two-week period. Sessions focus on behavior modification, goal setting, mastering obstacles, and social support. The American Cancer Society also publishes a free handbook for potential quitters, the *I Quit Kit*, which is available from your local chapter (consult your telephone directory for the address and phone number) or from their national headquarters at the address above.

The Breathe-Free Plan to Stop Smoking
Narcotics Education, Inc.
6830 Laurel Street, NW
Washington, DC 20012

Many local affiliates of the Seventh-Day Adventist Church run a highly recommended program that is usually led by a pastor-physician team. The Breathe-Free Plan to Stop Smoking is based on motivation, lifestyle modification, values clarification, modeling, visualization, affirmation, positive thinking, and self-rewards. There is also an optional nondenominational spiritual component.

The plan consists of eight sessions that take place over three weeks, with periodic phone contacts for one year thereafter. Prospective group members are invited to attend the first two sessions before making a decision as to whether to register for the remainder of the course. During the third week a graduation ceremony is held. Successful quitters receive a BNS (Bachelor of Nonsmoking) degree during the third week. MNS (Master of Nonsmoking) degrees are awarded at six months, and DNS (Doctor of Nonsmoking) degrees at twelve months.

Smokers Anonymous
P.O. Box 25335
West Los Angeles, CA 90025
(212) 474–8997

This group provides information on starting your own support group. They will also let you know if there is a Smokers Anonymous group in your area. Write to them at the above address, enclosing a self-addressed stamped envelope.

Rapid Smoking

Think back to your first cigarette. After the first few puffs you probably felt dizzy and sick to your stomach. It took you a long time to learn to tolerate a full lungful of smoke.

Rapid smoking is a clever and effective technique designed to make you more aware of those very unpleasant effects you have learned to tolerate. It thus helps make smoking less attractive, which in turn makes it easier to quit.

To practice rapid smoking, smokers allow themselves to smoke as many cigarettes as they wish—indeed, the more the better—but they must smoke them in a pre-scribed manner.

As there are some possible risks involving this proce-dure, rapid smoking should be used only under the supervision of a physician or as part of a professionally supervised smoking cessation clinic. Before using this method, review your health history with a physician or smoking cessation specialist to determine whether you are a good candidate for rapid smoking. If you have had a heart attack or have diabetes or a history of disease of the heart, lungs, or blood vessels, use this method only under a physician's direct supervision. If you suffer from congestive heart failure, if you are pregnant, or if you have not obtained a physician's approval, this technique should *not* be used.

Here is a set of guidelines used at one center.[4] Specific methods vary from center to center.

- While using this technique, avoid all smoking except during scheduled sessions.

- Pick one place in which you will practice rapid smok-ing. Choose a place free of distractions such as radio or TV, where you will be alone, undisturbed, and fac-ing a blank wall. Keep all windows closed. Turn off any fan, heater, or air conditioning.

- Schedule rapid smoking sessions in advance. Allow 30 minutes for each session.

- You will need the following supplies for each session:
    —two packs of cigarettes
    —matches
    —a candle

   —a large ashtray
   —a watch or clock with a second hand
   —a wastebasket or trash can with a plastic liner

- The average smoker takes a puff about every 30 to 90 seconds. In rapid smoking, you will take as large a puff as possible every 6 seconds.

- When the time for your session comes, go to your chosen place. Assemble your supplies on the table in front of you. Place the wastebasket on the floor beside you (this is to be used in case of vomiting). Light the candle. Then light the first cigarette. Remember to take a puff every 6 seconds. When you have finished the first cigarette, *immediately* light another from the candle flame. Continue until you begin to feel nauseated; *or* you cannot stand to smoke anymore; *or* you have smoked three cigarettes.

Rapid smoking has been extensively studied. Researchers Brian G. Danaher and Edward Lichtenstein conclude that "rapid smoking has received perhaps the most intensive investigation of any smoking-control procedure." It has consistently been found effective in studies by a wide variety of investigators. Studies show that one or more periods of rapid smoking shortly before quitting markedly increase smokers' chances of sustained success in quitting.

Effective as it may be, the rapid smoking technique is not a pleasant experience. Many researchers believe that it should be used only as a method of last resort, after other attempts to quit have failed.

Lichtenstein and Glasgow estimate that at least 35,000 smokers have used rapid smoking in various studies without serious ill effects. Even hard-core smokers with heart or lung disease can use this method, but only under the direct supervision of a physician.[5]

Using Audio and Video Tapes to Help You Quit

If you're one of the millions of busy people who enjoy listening to cassette tapes—or if you're a friend, family member, or professional interested in helping others quit—you'll be glad to know that the guilt-free, self-care approach to quitting espoused in *The No-Nag, No-Guilt, Do-It-Your-Own-Way Guide to Quitting Smoking* also serves as the guiding principle for a high-quality set of cassette tapes I recently developed and wrote for Syber-Vision Systems, one of the USA's leading producers of self-care audio and videotape packages. This eight-audiotape series, entitled *The Neuropsychology of Smoking Cessation: How to Quit Smoking for Life*, is organized around the ten stages of quitting described on pages 143–145 and 173–176. You, the smoker, listen to the entire set of cassettes in advance for an overview of the self-directed quitting process. You then go back and use each cassette repeatedly as you are passing through the stage it describes. As you successfully complete each stage of the quitting process, you move on to the cassette for the *new* stage you have just entered.

Each cassette is designed to be played repeatedly, to boost your motivation and to remind you of the key strategies you'll need to make it successfully through the particular stage you're in. The last cassette in the series is addressed to your spouse, other family members, and your closest friends. It instructs them to stop nagging you about your smoking and tells them exactly how to give you the encouragement, understanding, and support you'll need to help you through the quitting process.

The Neuropsychology of Smoking Cessation: How to Quit Smoking for Life can be ordered in two ways. You can purchase the complete eight-cassette audio program plus the study guide, *or* you can order the eight-cassette program, the study guide, plus *Quitting for Life*, a 30-minute support video.

Your truly (T.F.) appears on the video, talking you step by step through the ten stages of quitting. You can watch it anytime you feel a need for additional information and support. The video can also be used to demonstrate the essentials of this guilt-free, self-care approach to quitting for friends, family, or clients. It can also be used as a trigger tape for classes or workshops.

You can order the eight-cassette audio program plus the study guide for $69.95 postpaid. The 30-minute video, *Quitting for Life*, is $39.95 postpaid. Or order *both* the audiotape package *and* the video for only $89.95. To place your order, write the Center for Self-Care Studies, 3805 Stevenson Avenue, Austin TX 78703. For VISA or Mastercard orders, phone (512) 472-1333. All audio and video packages come with a 60-day money back guarantee. Rush delivery is available. When ordering the video, please specify VHS or Beta format. Discounts available on quantity orders.

Other Tips to Help You Quit

Several years ago, when we began the research for this book, we started running the following advertisement in *Medical SelfCare:*[6]

SMOKERS AND HEALTH—We're compiling a collection of self-care tips for health-concerned smokers and would welcome your suggestions on quitting, cutting down, and staying healthier while still smoking.

We received hundreds of suggestions. Many have been included throughout *The No-Nag, No-Guilt Do-It-Your-Own-Way Guide to Quitting Smoking*. Many thanks to all the *Medical SelfCare* readers who took the time and trouble to send us their favorite tips. Below we offer a roundup of some of the best tips.

KEEP YOUR HANDS BUSY

"Make it a game to collect all the nonsmoking things you can to keep your hands busy: Knit a sweater. Write letters. Do crosswords. Read a book. Polish your glasses. Chew a toothpick. Crack your knuckles. Do puzzles. The best one of all for me was to take up drawing. (A wonderful do-it-yourself drawing guide is *Drawing on the Left Side of the Brain* by Betty Edwards.)"

THE EPICUREAN METHOD

"I found it relatively easy to quit after cutting down to one extremely expensive imported Turkish cigarette per day. I bought them one at a time for 50 cents each, and I never allowed myself to buy more than one. I'd keep it on a special shelf in the dining room and would smoke it after dinner. I kept that up for three months, then the whole thing became too much of a hassle, so I quit."

FREQUENT SHOWERS

"Whenever you feel like a cigarette, take a long, hot shower instead. You may turn into a prune and run up a big water bill, but you'll stop smoking."

THIS ONE WILL KEEP YOUR SPOUSE HAPPY

"Keep a list of household chores (e.g., clean out kitchen drawers, wash the dog, put drain cleaner in the drains, regrout the tub, pull the weeds, mow the lawn). Every time you feel an urge to smoke, pick one chore from the list and do it.''

HAVE NONSMOKING FRIENDS TELL YOU THE TRUTH ON TAPE

''Have several nonsmoking friends who love you but hate your smoking make a tape in which they describe how disgusting your smoking is for them, then plead with you to quit. Listen to the tape first thing in the morning and just before you go to bed.''

CLOVE OIL

''Anytime you get the urge to smoke, put a drop of clove oil on your finger and apply it to the back of your tongue. It works like magic. You can buy clove oil in most natural food stores.''

LICORICE STICKS

''My husband recently quit smoking. The thing that really made the first month or so bearable was chewing on licorice sticks—not the candy, but actual licorice twigs, which he bought at our natural foods store. They have a pleasant taste and give you something to do with your hands and mouth. After three or four weeks, he found that he no longer needed them.''

VISIT THE CANCER WARD

"A physician friend of mine took me along to the hospital and introduced me to two of his patients, one with lung cancer and one with emphysema. I quit the next day."

CRITICIZING CIGARETTE ADS

"Criticize each cigarette ad you see. Let yourself realize that such ads are part of a cynical attempt to manipulate your behavior and put your dollars in the pockets of tobacco companies. Each time you see such an ad, think of what these brands might be called if these ads really told the truth: e.g., Unlucky Strikes, Halitosis 100's, Fools, Pale Male, Emphysema Slims, etc."

WILLIE AND MERLE

"Get a copy of the song 'Reasons to Quit,' sung by Willie Nelson and Merle Haggard—it's on their album *Pancho and Lefty*. Make a tape that contains only that one song, played over and over again. Don't play any other records or tapes until you really *do* quit."

ONE STEP AT A TIME

"I succeeded in quitting by taking it one step at a time: First I stopped smoking in my car. Then in my house. Then at the office. Then before breakfast. I just nickeled and dimed away at it until I eliminated every single smoking situation except one—standing on a busy corner six blocks from my house after dinner. And that was so incovenient I finally just said to hell with it."

TESTING YOUR SENSE OF SMELL

"Here's a simple test to show you how much of the sense of smell you've lost because of your smoking: Close your eyes. Have a friend take a cigarette and hold it at various distances from your nose. See how far away it is when you can just barely smell it. Now repeat the same test with a nonsmoking friend. The friend's sense of smell will be much more sensitive."

AVOID H.A.L.T.

"In my stop-smoking program they warned us to avoid H.A.L.T. after we quit—that is, avoid becoming too Hungry, too Angry, too Lonely, or too Tired. I found it valuable advice indeed."

SUNFLOWER SEEDS

"Buy a couple of pounds of sunflower seeds. Put a small quantity in a number of little plastic bags and stash them around in your house, car, office, purse, etc. When you have an urge to light up, reach for a handful of sunflower seeds instead."

LIMITING ALCOHOL INTAKE

"The key to my successful quitting was limiting my alcohol intake to one glass of beer or wine a day, with meals. I'd tried to quit several times before, but had always ended up having a cigarette after a few drinks."

BRUSHING TEETH AFTER MEALS

"My Achilles' heel when it came to cigarettes was the time when I'd be sitting around relaxing after a good meal. I found it worked really well for me to jump up as soon as I finished eating, go into the bathroom, and spend a good five or ten minutes brushing and flossing my teeth.''

MORE MOZART

''I quit by setting aside enough money to buy myself a new Mozart album every day for the first ten days, then one a week for the next ten weeks. Whenever I got an urge to smoke, I'd go listen to Mozart instead.''

REFRIGERATOR PHOTOS

''Have a friend take pictures of you smoking, really ugly ones. Have them take a whole bunch, then pick out the ones that are absolutely the worst. Have them enlarged and put them on your refrigerator. When you're tempted to smoke, look at the picture and remember how 'glamorous' it makes you look. After you've gone without smoking for three months, you can take the pictures down.''

FILLING THE URGE WITH WHAT'S THERE

''My meditation teacher gave me some advice that was extremely useful in helping me quit. He said, 'When you feel the urge to smoke, acknowledge the urge, consider it a request, then find a way to fill that request with whatever happens to be right in front of you.' This has proved to be an invaluable bit of advice, not only for smoking, but in many other areas of my life.''

Daily Cigarette Log

Daily Cigarette Log for_____

No.	Time	Place/Activity	With Whom	Mood	Urge
1.					
2.					
3.					
4.					
5.					
6.					
7.					
8.					
9.					
10.					
11.					
12.					
13.					
14.					
15.					
16.					
17.					
18.					
19.					
20.					
21.					
22.					
23.					
24.					
25.					
26.					
27.					
28.					
29.					
30.					
31.					
32.					
33.					
34.					
35.					
36.					
37.					
38.					
39.					
40.					

Contract to Quit Smoking

I,_____ , do hearby solemnly swear to quit smoking forever. My quitting date will be_____ .

Between now and my quitting date, I will observe my smoking behavior, experiment with alternatives, record my urges and number of cigarettes smoked, and keep a smoking journal. During this time I will work daily to change my smoking-related thought patterns and to reduce my intake of tobacco smoke. On the day I have chosen, I will stop smoking forever.

_____   _____
Name   Date

In witness whereof:

_____   _____
Support Person   Date

11
Dealing with Weight Gain

The smokers we interviewed told us that fear of weight gain was a major barrier to quitting. Many rated it as their number one barrier. Several flatly stated that they would not attempt to quit because of their concerns about weight gain.

Weight-related concerns about quitting seem to be especially great for women. This special concern is due, in part, to cultural factors: Women are "expected" to be thin. It may also be that women smokers who quit are at higher risk for weight gain: Some animal studies suggest that the weight-controlling effects of nicotine are greater in females.[1]

Do Smokers Weigh Less?

The fact is that many, but not all, ex-smokers do gain some weight after they quit. One study found that 60 percent of men and 51 percent of women ex-smokers put on extra pounds. The average long-term weight gain for quitters is about 5 pounds, although some ex-smokers gain 20 pounds or more. Heavy smokers (40 or more cigarettes per day) who quit typically gain more weight than those who smoke fewer cigarettes. And young quitters show smaller weight gains than their older counterparts.[2] But these are *average* figures. It is only those who watch their food intake *carefully* who don't put on the pounds after quitting.[3]

Although many quitters do put on some weight, a sizable minority do not. A study at the University of California School of Medicine in San Francisco found that while 47 percent of long-term quitters gained 5 pounds or more and 30 percent gained 0–4 pounds, 23 percent actually *lost* weight.

The Risk of Being Overweight vs. The Risk of Smoking

Some prospective quitters worry that the possible weight gain they experience after quitting may be a greater health risk than their present smoking habit. This is an unrealistic concern for most smokers. The degree of weight gain is relatively small in most cases. To reach the same health risk as smoking one pack of cigarettes per day, the average smoker would have to be roughly 125 pounds overweight.[4]

Why Ex-smokers Gain Weight

Smokers weigh less because smoking depresses the appetite for certain foods, while quitters, whose appetites are not suppressed, gain weight because they take in more calories. While food intake may not be the only factor operating—nicotine may also alter the smoker's metabolism so that smokers burn more calories and convert fewer calories into fat[5]—food intake *and* increased exercise levels are clearly the major controllable factors in avoiding weight gain.

The "Sweet Tooth Factor"

A landmark study by psychologist Neil E. Grunberg of the Uniformed Services University of the Health Sciences, Bethesda, Maryland, has shed new light on this question. Grunberg was intrigued by earlier work that suggested that when subjects were given a dish of gumdrops and allowed to eat all they wanted, both nonsmokers and deprived smokers consumed more gumdrops than smokers. He wondered if nicotine could affect a person's consumption of sweet foods without affecting consumption of nonsweet foods.

He set up two experiments to find out: The first was done with rats. Grunberg found that when the rats were given high levels of nicotine, they ate fewer sweets. As a result they did not gain as much weight as other rats. When the nicotine was stopped, they again consumed more sweets—and put on weight as a result. There was no change in the rats' consumption of nonsweet foods during or after nicotine administration.

The second experiment used three groups of human volunteers—nonsmokers, smokers forbidden to smoke, and smokers who were allowed to smoke freely before the experiment. Each subject was asked to sample nine different foods. Three of the foods were sweet (chocolate, coffee cake, gumdrops), three were salty (salami, salted peanuts, pretzels), and three were bland (unsalted crackers, cheese, unsalted peanuts). After they had tasted all nine foods, the subjects were left alone in the room and were told to eat as much as they wanted of each food.

After they left, the bowls were weighed and the consumption of each food was recorded.

The most striking difference between the consumption patterns of the three groups was that *smokers ate a far smaller amount of sweet food than nonsmokers.* The deprived smokers ate an intermediate amount. Dr. Grunberg concluded that smoking appears to decrease the appetite for sweet foods. He speculates that this may be because nicotine triggers a change in glucose availability in the body.[6]

How Smoking Changes Your Metabolism

Smoking also appears to affect digestion. When smoking researcher Ellen Gritz of UCLA did a study of stomach emptying in smokers and nonsmokers she found that food remained in the smokers' stomach considerably longer. Fullness of the stomach is thought to signal the brain that one should stop eating. Thus, this could be one of the ways that smoking tends to reduce smokers' body weight.[7] Other studies suggest that smokers may burn more calories.[8]

In addition, smoking:

- provides the smoker with a substitute activity for eating;

- increases the passage of food through the lower digestive tract by increasing the propulsive activity of the colon. Thus, some food may be swept through before all nutrients are absorbed;

- serves as a marker of meal termination. Rather than taking a second or third helping or having dessert, smokers are likely to stop eating and have a cigarette.

All these factors, considered together, may help explain why smokers can lose weight while nonsmokers who take in the same number of calories may gain weight.

Why Some Quitters *Don't* Gain Weight

Recent studies of certain enzymes in our fat cells suggest that the reason some smokers gain weight after quitting while others do not may be in part a matter of genetics. One of the key enzymes in the regulation of fat storage is lipoprotein lipase. This enzyme breaks down circulating triglycerides, liberating free fatty acids that can then be taken up and stored by the fat cells. High activity levels of this enzyme are thought to increase the efficiency of fat storage, and thus to produce weight gain. Low levels are thought to produce less efficient energy storage, and thus to promote weight loss. Researchers believe that genetic differences account for high or low levels of lipoprotein lipase in different people.

A recent study by researchers Robert M. Carney of the Washington University School of Medicine in St. Louis and Andrew P. Goldberg of the Baltimore City Hospital found that smokers with high levels of lipoprotein lipase gained more weight after they quit, while smokers with the lowest levels of this enzyme actually lost weight after quitting.

The researchers concluded that a test that measured lipoprotein lipase activity might help predict a smoker's potential for weight gain after quitting. This test is not currently available.[9]

Lung Damage and Weight Loss

Another factor contributing to lower body weight in smokers could be impaired lung function. Recent studies by B. Nemery and his colleagues suggest that it is only those smokers with the most extensive smoking-produced lung damage who exhibit marked weight loss. The researchers found that smokers with normal lung function weighed roughly the same as nonsmokers.[10]

Munching as an Effective Quit-Smoking Strategy

Another recent study found that smokers who consumed more food or liquids, or avoided other cigarette-associated substances such as alcohol and coffee, were more successful in cutting down their smoking than subjects who attempted to reduce smoking with no specific plan. The researchers concluded that weight gain following quitting may be due, in part, to the fact that the quitters are using eating as a substitute for smoking.[11]

Exercise Can Help Prevent Weight Gain

None of the studies listed above took exercise status into account. When University of Minnesota Researchers David R. Jacobs and Sara Gottenborg looked at the effects of both smoking status and exercise level, they found that the weight gain attributed to smoking was roughly equal to the weight loss attributed to an active lifestyle.

Jacobs and Gottenborg's research suggests that the weight-lowering effects of an active lifestyle are slightly greater for men (11 pounds) than for women (7 pounds). The weight difference between light to moderate smokers and ex-smokers was about 9 pounds for both men and women.[12]

Strategy #1: Ignore Weight Gain

What is a prospective quitter to make of all this? One very popular approach—perhaps the most common—is just to go ahead and quit. After all, you may be one of the lucky ones who gains little or no weight. This is a particularly reasonable approach for light smokers and those who would not be greatly upset by gaining a few pounds.

If you decide to take this approach, go ahead and get yourself permanently separated from cigarettes. Then review the situation and decide what you will do about it. *Warning:* This approach is not recommended if the prospect of gaining weight is so unacceptable to you that a small weight gain might result in a relapse.

Strategy #2: Use Exercise To Control Weight

The smokers we interviewed told us that it is difficult indeed to quit smoking and to try to make other major lifestyle changes at the same time. They warn that quitting will take all your available energy and efforts. Thus, other major life changes should be instituted either before or after you quit.

This is especially true for exercise. The best way to use exercise to help control weight after quitting might be to begin a regular exercise program several months *before* your planned quitting date.

There are many advantages to this approach. Not only will exercise help keep your weight down, it can also (as we saw in chapter 5) make it easier for you to quit and will provide you with an alternative activity that will help you make it through the most difficult parts of cigarette withdrawal.

One successful quitter, Roger, used the following method:

"I'd tried and failed to quit several times. One of the things that always bothered me was that I'd immediately start to gain weight. So this time, before I tried again, I decided to start exercising.

"I'm a morning person, so I decided I'd go out for a brisk walk every day, right after I got up. I went through my calendar for three months in advance and scheduled myself for six exercise sessions per week, from six-thirty to seven every weekday morning and at whatever time I felt like getting up on Saturday.

"I allowed myself some built-in flexibility by giving myself permission to 'cheat' by skipping one, *but only one*, walking session per week. I usually tried not to miss a single day during the week so I could take Saturday off. But I'd almost always go out on Saturday anyway if the weather was good.

"I started out slow and gradually increased my speed. I bought myself a good pair of walking shoes and a headset radio so I could listen to the morning news. I eventually bought myself a running outfit and a rain hat so I could walk in any weather.

"After the first month I really began to feel better. It got easier and easier to pass on having a cigarette. By the end of two months I'd lost four pounds. I was so excited I increased my sessions to 45 minutes per day. By the end of three months, I'd cut down from over a pack a day to eight cigarettes per day. One day as I was coming home from my walk I decided, 'O.K. I'm ready. I'm going to go for it.'

"The day I quit I started walking for a full hour every morning. For the first few weeks, I did a lot of walking in the evenings as well. My wife is definitely *not* a morning person. It was a lot easier to get her to go out with me in the evening. I did a lot of walking that first, difficult week. When I felt an especially strong urge to smoke, I went outside and walked around the block until it passed.

"I did gain a couple of pounds after I quit, but since I'd already lost a few, I figure I came out about even. I probably *would* gain weight if I quit walking, but I've really gotten to like it, so I'm not about to stop. I figure I could probably lose *more* weight by walking more, but I'm pretty happy right where I am."

Strategy #3: The Sugarfree Solution

As with exercise, it's difficult indeed to quit smoking and to change your eating patterns at the same time. The best guideline here seems to be to start taking control of your eating *before* you quit.

Neil Grunberg's study, described above, suggests that smokers who quit needn't go on a full-scale, all-out diet. Instead, they should restrict the type, but not the quantity, of food in their environment. Grunberg suggests that ex-smokers can ease their craving for sweets by using sugar substitutes or eating fruit. This need only be a temporary measure. Your extra urge for sweets will fade as your body readjusts its blood sugar level.[13]

Here are some good foods to stock up on:

• fruit juices
• sunflower seeds

- spring or mineral water
- carrots
- popcorn (without butter)
- yogurt (low-fat, unsweetened)
- V-8 juice
- apples
- bananas
- dry-roasted peanuts

Mealtime Solutions

Pay special attention to your mealtime routine during your pre-quitting and quitting efforts. Many prospective quitters have been dismayed to discover that whereas they had previously left the table early to have a cigarette, once they quit they find themselves remaining at the table for second or third helpings. Here are some mealtime tips to help ex-smokers watch their weight:

- Take smaller portions. (One way to encourage yourself to do this is to use a smaller plate.)

- Eat slowly. Try to be the last one done.

- Take smaller bites. Chew and swallow each bite before taking the next. Become aware of the taste and texture of your food.

- Put your fork down between mouthfuls.

- Pour yourself a large glass of ice water with every meal. Take frequent sips between bites.

- Have a family member prepare your portions and put extra food away so that seconds are not easily accessible.

- Serve sliced fruit for dessert—or skip dessert altogether.

- As soon as you finish, get up from the table.

- Pick a nonsmoking activity to be a sign of meal termination. Take a walk, brush your teeth, wash the dishes, take a shower, puff on a plastic cigarette, eat an artificially sweetened mint, or develop your own meal termination ritual.[14]

Between-Meal Solutions

Recent quitters frequently experience strong urges to snack or to have something in their mouths. If sweets are available you may feel a powerful urge to nibble. You may also feel an urge to hold something in place of a cigarette. Here are some tips to help you avoid overdoing it on high-sugar snacks:

- Allow yourself unlimited amounts of raw vegetables: carrot or celery sticks, cherry tomatoes, cucumber slices, broccoli flowerets, cauliflower buds, etc. Keep these in the front of the refrigerator, where they are easily accessible.

- Always carry a good supply of sugarless gum, mints, and candy. Eat only one piece of candy or gum at a time and try to make each piece last as long as possible.

- Allow yourself moderate amounts of such low-calorie snacks as bread sticks, Rykrisp, unbuttered popcorn, pretzels, etc. Avoid snacks that contain large amounts of sugar or fat.

- Stay away from alcohol. Alcoholic beverages are high in calories. In addition, alcohol can produce breakdowns in self-control that may lead to eating binges or a smoking-relapse crisis.

- Unshelled sunflower seeds or unshelled peanuts are particularly good snacks. They occupy both hands and mouth and the process of removing the shells slows down consumption.

- Allow no high-calorie snacks in the house for three to six months after you quit. If this is not possible, seal high-calorie snacks in plastic bags and put them in a hard-to-reach cupboard.

- Ask friends and family not to offer you food.

- When you feel the urge to snack, go for a walk instead.

- During the early stages of quitting, avoid parties where high-calorie snacks will be served.

- Take healthy snacks with you when you will be away from home.

- Go to bed earlier than usual to avoid the temptation to snack.

- Keep yourself occupied with puzzles, knitting, gardening, creative crafts, housework, home repairs, etc.

Tips for Keeping Your Weight Down After You Quit

- If possible, don't set your quitting date shortly before holidays when it is customary to consume high-calorie food and drinks. The temptation to munch may be too hard to resist.

- Weight Watchers or similar groups can be a big help in your efforts to control your weight. The best time to join such a group is *before* you quit.

- Weigh yourself daily, at the same time every day. Record your daily weight on a chart or calendar. This will make you more aware of weight changes.

- Develop your own alternative activities or rituals to use when you feel the urge for a cigarette. One successful quitter installed water coolers both at home and at his office. Whenever he felt the urge for a cigarette, he would simply go to the cooler and drink a glass of chilled spring water. Other smokers adopt a special drink—iced tea, iced coffee, or a favorite diet soda— as their alternative of choice.

- Liza, an ex-smoker we interviewed, came up with a unique approach to the weight-control problem: "When I quit smoking I gained twelve pounds. I was determined to lose it. I decided I wanted to kick off my weight-loss program by doing something dramatic. I drove to a supermarket two miles from my house, marched up to the butcher counter, and had them grind me twelve pounds of fresh hamburger. I left my car in the parking lot and carried it home.

  "By the time I got home, I was exhausted. Twelve pounds is a *lot* of hamburger. Twelve pounds of excess fat is a heavy load too, yet I was carrying that much extra weight around with me every day. No wonder I felt tired all the time.

  "I gave most of the hamburger away to friends and neighbors. The very next day I started running every afternoon. I became very picky about what I ate. I did succeed in shedding those twelve pounds. It took about six months. But it all started that afternoon I walked home with twelve pounds of hamburger in my arms."

Realistic Goals for Weight Control

The problem of smoking and its effect on weight control can be a particularly difficult one for people who feel that they have a weight problem even *with* smoking. Humorist Alice Kahn recently proposed that those struggling with extra poundage adopt what she calls the All New Feminist No-Weight-Loss Diet: Stop trying to lose weight, eat whatever you want, and accept your rightful place in the Heavy Majority.

Although Kahn was writing with tongue in cheek, a modified version of her prescription is certainly worth considering. For smokers who wish to quit but aren't willing to exercise and prefer not to make changes in their eating patterns, the wisest course may well be to go ahead and let yourself gain a few pounds. Recent studies suggest that except for diabetics and people with high blood pressure, earlier claims made for the health benefits of losing a few extra pounds have been considerably exaggerated.

The urge to be slim is so widespread in our culture that it is rarely questioned. As Kahn writes, "Fatness has become our number one socially unacceptable physical trait. Dr. Margaret MacKenzie of the University of California, who has compared attitudes toward fat in the U.S. and Samoa, calls the prevalent American view 'the new racism.' In her view, holistic health and 'new age' groups are among the most militant fat-phobes. Thinness is viewed not only as healthier, but also as politically correct."[15]

Some researchers have begun to question our culture's fat phobia. Kim Chernin, author of *The Obsession: Reflections on the Tyranny of Slenderness*[16] refers to our culture's demand that women be slim as "the women's reduction movement." She compares it to the practice of foot binding in parts of Asia.

It has long been taken for granted that being overweight is simply due to overeating, but recent research suggests that the matter is much more complex than this.

There is growing evidence that each of us may be biochemically programmed for a certain weight, our so-called setpoint. While it may be possible to keep ourselves temporarily below our setpoint through crash diets, in the long run we will almost inevitably drift back to our setpoints.

Many researchers now believe that the very idea of "going on a diet" dooms the prospective dieter to failure. The typical dieter believes that she will go through a brief period of eating less than adequate portions of "diet foods" she doesn't really like in order to lose a few pounds. However, these foods and these portions are *not* what she's planning to eat for the rest of her life. Unfortunately, she soon reverts to her former eating style and goes right back to her former weight.

In the long run, dieting appears to alter one's metabolism in a way that actually *interferes* with weight loss—probably by affecting the activity level of certain fat-storage enzymes. Diets can also create food-anxiety that may lead to later binge eating.[17]

In certain cases, people who are overweight can get some insight into emotional and psychological reasons that led them to eat by keeping an eating journal in which they record everything they eat as well as how they are feeling and what is going on in their lives. One ex-smoker we interviewed realized that she was undermining her efforts to quit. Because she felt irritable while going through withdrawal, she frequently found herself picking a fight with her husband. Afterward, she'd run to the refrigerator and eat to console herself. She would then use the resulting weight gain as an excuse to give up her quitting efforts.

In addition to helping prospective quitters become fully aware of the emotional chains that bind them to the refrigerator door, an eating journal provides an excellent alternative activity—when you feel hungry, instead of eating, you can *write* about eating. If you find that you have a deep resistance to the idea of exercising, you can write about that too.

12

How to *Stay* a Nonsmoker: Quitting as an Adult Life Transition

Over 1,000 Americans a day die of smoking-related disease. Quitting reduces or eliminates all of smoking's harmful effects. Yet all too many who quit return to smoking. As Mark Twain said, "Quitting smoking is easy. I've done it hundreds of times."

While quitting is a necessary step, it is only the *first* step on a long journey. In making this journey, the new ex-smoker will encounter a long succession of potential relapse crisis situations. The next challenge is to *remain* a nonsmoker. And the key skills required for remaining a nonsmoker are the skills of *relapse prevention*.[1]

The Two Commandments of Relapse Prevention

In order for a relapse to occur, three things must happen: (1) The new ex-smoker must be presented with a potential relapse crisis situation; (2) the relapse crisis situation must trigger an intense cigarette craving; (3) the craving must overwhelm the ex-smoker's ability to cope. To avoid relapse, the new ex-smoker must identify every potential relapse crisis situation at the earliest possible moment and must choose an effective coping strategy and put it into action immediately.

The idea that one must identify each high-risk situation and respond with an appropriate coping strategy lies at the very heart of successful quitting. All the tips and tools, all the pharmacology and pro-health strategies notwithstanding, it is how you deal with a potential relapse crisis that will determine whether or not you will become a permanent nonsmoker. If you identify each potential crisis and respond appropriately, you'll succeed. If you don't, you'll fail. It's as simple as that.

Troubleshooting a Relapse Crisis

Let's follow a typical new quitter as she encounters her first serious relapse crisis. Cathy has made it through her first week as a nonsmoker. She feels that she has come through the worst of it, and believes she deserves to reward herself for sticking it out so long. She offers to take her fiancé, Peter, out to dinner and a movie to celebrate.

She and Peter go to a fancy restaurant and have a lovely dinner—complete with a bottle of good California Chardonnay. As they're finishing their coffee and brandy, Cathy's boss and his wife come over to say hello. They bring their drinks with them. It is only after they have sat down and begun talking that the boss's wife lights a cigarette.

Right away, warning signals go off in Cathy's brain. The smell of the smoke triggers a powerful urge: She can't believe how much she wants a cigarette. She realizes, with horror, that she is beginning to offer herself rationalizations: "One little cigarette won't hurt."

"You've been so good—you deserve a reward." She is exhausted and frustrated after her first difficult week as a nonsmoker. And she realizes that the wine, the brandy, and the good meal have put her in an extremely vulnerable position. The waitress comes over. The boss and his wife order more drinks and invite Cathy and Peter to join them.

Cathy understands that she is face to face with a serious relapse crisis. She is faced with a problem in what smoking researcher Saul Shiffman and his colleagues call *meta-coping*—deciding which coping response to use.[2]

Fortunately, Cathy recognizes the danger and is able to come up with an appropriate response. She declines gracefully, explaining that she and Peter need to leave immediately if they are to make their movie. She stands up, explaining that the dinner is her treat and she must go to the cashier's desk to ask about something on the bill. She waits there until Peter says goodbye and joins her. On their way out she explains her action. Peter, who has been serving as her principal support person for quitting, is sympathetic and understanding.

When faced with a smoking relapse situation, the ex-smoker who does not act quickly is unlikely to be effective in resisting temptation. Situations that increase the chances of failure include those in which the ex-smoker has been eating or drinking; is feeling depressed or angry; takes too long to begin a coping response; or chooses an inadequate response. In addition, high levels of stress or interpersonal conflict, as well as the presence of smokers or smoking paraphernalia at social gatherings where there is social pressure to smoke increase the chance of a relapse.[3]

Potential Relapse Crisis Situations[17]

Read through each of the following scenarios, imagining that you have recently quit and now find yourself in the situation described. On a scale of 1 to 10, rate the intensity of the urge to smoke that would result from each situation (1 representing a very mild urge for a cigarette, 10 representing an almost overpowering urge to smoke).

1. You've just picked up your car from the mechanic and the bill is twice as much as you expected. As you drive home you find that the very problem you took the car in for is *still* not fixed. As a result, the car stalls in rush-hour traffic. You feel angry and frustrated. You open the glove compartment to consult the owner's manual and discover a forgotten pack of cigarettes. You find that you *really* want one.

2. You're sitting on the back patio with a few friends on a balmy evening, sipping a cool beer and enjoying the company. One of your friends lights a cigarette and offers you one. It smells wonderful.

3. You're on your way home from work feeling tired, hungry, and depressed. You stop at the supermarket, fill a cart with groceries, then discover that you've forgotten to bring any money. On your way out of the store a friendly salesclerk offers you a free sample of a new brand of cigarettes.

4. You're at home alone on a Sunday evening, feeling bored and blue. You can't think of a thing in the world that would be the least bit interesting—except going out and getting a cigarette.

5. You're at a party with friends and have had several glasses of wine. Everyone else seems to be smoking. You remember how satisfying it used to be. You *still* can't figure out what to do with your hands at a party without a cigarette to hold. A friend offers you a cigarette—your old brand. It sure looks appealing.

6. You've been working under pressure all day. The phone has been ringing off the hook, keeping you from getting anything done, and your boss bawled you out for something that wasn't your fault. A coworker stopped by to discuss the rumor of impending layoffs. You realize that your job may be affected. When you finally get home, you find you can't relax. It occurs to you that a cigarette might help.

7. You're driving with one of your oldest friends. He's complaining that your decision to quit has driven a wedge into the very heart of your friendship. He feels abandoned because you no longer smoke with him and you act so uncomfortable when he lights up. That reminds him that he is completely out of cigarettes. He pulls over at a corner store and asks you to run in and buy him a pack while he drives around the block. You come out of the store with the cigarettes and a pack of matches, remembering all the times your friend has been there for you in the past. As you stand waiting for him, you have a tremendous urge to light up a cigarette and to be smoking it when he arrives.

8. You've had a serious fight with your spouse. You realize, for the first time, that your marriage may not survive. You remember that a friend recently left a pack of cigarettes behind. They're in the kitchen drawer, just waiting for you. You need one badly. It seems fated that you should have one. After all, nothing else in your life seems to be working.

9. Your boss has been pressuring you to finish the project you're working on. The office is a madhouse and you're having trouble concentrating. You know that things will only get worse later in the day. You're sure a cigarette would help you concentrate long enough to get the job done.

10. Some good friends have just lost a child to an auto accident. You try to comfort them as best you can, and because they're in such pain, you don't mention that you are quitting. Unfortunately, they're both heavy smokers. You don't feel comfortable asking them not to smoke in their own home, it wouldn't be right to leave, and you *know* if you stay there another second, you're going to have to have a cigarette yourself.

Now go back through the list and think of at least three effective coping responses you could use in each situation.

Two Types of Coping Responses

Successful coping responses include both internal responses (things you might think) and active responses (things you might do).[4] In the above situation, Cathy chose an active response—she simply excused herself and left the scene of the potential relapse situation. Other active measures might have included mentioning the fact that she had quit, asking the boss's wife if she would mind putting out her cigarette, or chewing a piece of nicotine gum. Cathy might also have chosen an internal response: imagining a smoker's lung ravaged by cancer; reminding herself how much she liked the fact that her clothes no longer smelled of smoke; or giving herself a verbal command that she was *not* going to have a cigarette.

Active and Internal Coping Responses[18]

Active Responses—Things You Might Do

- Have something to eat.
- Choose a nonalcoholic drink.
- Engage in physical exercise.
- Engage in sex.
- Take several deep, slow breaths.
- Find something to occupy your hands (a puzzle, knitting, a book).
- Avoid social gatherings where there will be drinking and smoking.
- Talk to a friend about quitting.
- Take a hot bath or shower.
- Write a letter to someone you love, telling them about your experience of quitting.

Internal Responses—Things You Might Think

- Think about the positive benefits of not smoking (health, pride, etc.).
- Think about the negative effects of smoking (disease, death, smelly clothes, etc.).
- Give yourself commands (''Don't do it!'' ''Stop!'' ''You will *not* smoke!'').
- Remind yourself how hard it was to quit in the first place.
- Tell yourself you really *don't* want to smoke.
- Distract yourself by thinking about other things.
- Imagine the immediate harmful effects of smoking (black lungs, carbon monoxide in your blood, etc.).
- Tell yourself you only need to keep from smoking one day at a time.
- Acknowledge the difficulty of quitting and praise yourself for taking on this challenge.
- Imagine yourself a successful ex-smoker, celebrating your first full year without using tobacco.

Why Smokers *Start* Smoking

Smokers typically take up the cigarette habit as teenagers. They do so not out of an innate enjoyment of their first few puffs, but out of a desire to be accepted by a particular social group and to be more comfortable in social interactions with other smokers. Smoking also provides important symbolic rewards; it is seen as both ''adult'' and ''forbidden.''

Without such pressures and rewards, it is unlikely that anyone would ever take up the habit at all. In the beginning, every novice smoker feels a physical revulsion to the toxic effect of tobacco smoke. If the social pressure and symbolic rewards are sustained, however, the apprentice smoker can eventually learn to tolerate these unpleasant effects.[5] And once smokers become physically addicted, it becomes difficult to stop.

To many young smokers, health concerns are of little

importance. Most teenagers perceive themselves as having a virtually inexhaustible supply of good health. The urge to conserve their health is less pressing than the need to demonstrate their independence by separating themselves from their parents and bonding with their peers. They feel they can afford to live dangerously: Health is something for older people to worry about. And at the age of fifteen or sixteen, "older people" applies to anyone over thirty.

Early adulthood, too, is a time of escaping from the limitations of childhood. It is a time of illusions and fantasies, of insecurities and stress. There is an overwhelming drive to become the person one was "meant" to be. Aspirations are high and accomplishments are as yet rather few. This is a period of striving with enthusiasm and discipline toward valued goals—educational and career success, testing one's ability to love and be loved, forming a long-term couple bond, raising a child, cementing one's professional identity, and achieving acceptance in the adult world.

During the early adult phase (from the late teens to the early or mid-thirties), smoking also plays an important role. It is used by some as a tool for increased self-control and self-regulation. It can help the young adult deal with stressful situations. It can serve as an instrument of social bonding. A cigarette may be used as a way to relax. Compared to these powerful and immediate benefits, the acknowledged but distant negative health effects may be only a nagging worry in the back of one's mind.

The Midlife Transition

But there comes a time for all of us when the effects of age begin to be felt. Like it or not, we must accept the fact that we have not been endowed with endless supplies of mental and physical energy. There comes a time when the abilities and reserves we have always relied on can be taken for granted no longer.

We become acutely aware that people in the generations ahead of us are growing ill or dying. We suddenly understand, with a depth of feeling we have never known before, that *we* are going to die, and that it will not be too many years until this occurs. We realize that we have been living our lives as if our own personal future stretched out forever. We now realize that the future is limited.

We become aware of a desperate urge to live our lives in such a way as to give meaning to the years to come. We begin, increasingly, to think of our health as something to be earned, conserved, and taken care of.[6]

For smokers, it is even harder to ignore the inescapable conclusion that our good health will not last forever. There comes a time when smokers can no longer deny that they have more wrinkles and less endurance than their nonsmoking fellows. They become increasingly aware of burned clothing and stained fingers and teeth. They realize that increasing numbers of their nonsmoking friends are disturbed by their smoking. Those who are parents may find their own children hostile to their use of tobacco.

Those who continue smoking become increasingly aware of the price they pay for every puff. The combination of the decline in health imposed by age and that imposed by smoking can become an immense and unwelcome burden. Many smokers, finally, reach the point where the price they are paying for their habit is too high.

Benefits vs. Drawbacks

If we would chart the perceived benefits and drawbacks of smoking in a typical smoker's life, we might see something like the following:

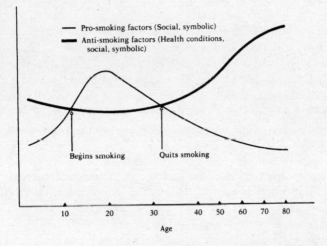

Figure 12-1 Perceived Advantages and Drawbacks of Smoking vs. Age[7]

For most of the smokers we interviewed, the perceived benefits of smoking increased rapidly during the middle and late teens, peaked in the mid-twenties, then dropped off rapidly thereafter. At the same time, the perceived drawbacks of smoking rose rapidly from about age thirty. It is the smoker who believes that the negative effects of smoking outweigh the benefits, yet who continues to smoke, who is most devilishly plagued by the self-recrimination and self-contempt we found among so many of the smokers we interviewed. For some smokers, the perceived benefits of smoking may be greater than the perceived drawbacks until well into later life, but the curve above represents the experience of the majority of the smokers and ex-smokers we interviewed.

Coming to Terms

The midlife transition is a time when one must come to terms with one's past and prepare for one's future. Many men and women who reach this stage of life find that they have a strong urge to review what they have done with their life thus far and to plan what they wish to do with the years ahead. For many, an important part of this reappraisal is deciding whether they wish to continue smoking.

For some, this period is characterized by struggles within the self and between the self and the external world. In his study of men going through the midlife transition, Daniel Levinson and his colleagues found that that was a time of moderate or severe crisis for 80 percent of their subjects.

Levinson and his colleagues feel that although the midlife transition may include some disruptive experiences, it is best understood as a normal and healthy developmental stage. The urge to question and modify one's life comes from the healthiest part of the self. As Levinson writes, one "can come to know, more than ever before, that powerful forces of destructiveness and creativity coexist in the human soul—in my soul!—and can integrate them in new ways."[8]

Most of the successful quitters we interviewed said that they saw quitting as part of a major and healthy life transition. Although outsiders sometimes saw them as "upset" or "sick," they themselves felt that they were going through a very positive transformation.

Dealing with Illusions

In attempting to reappraise one's life, the person in mid-life transition begins to become more conscious of those areas of life that have been shrouded in illusion and dominated by unconscious forces. Levinson calls this process of growing self-insight *de-illusionment*. He explains: "By this expression I mean a reduction of illusions, a recognition that long-held assumptions and beliefs about self and world are not true. . . . While playful illusions can be accepted as part of the imaginative world of childhood, an adult is expected to be more realistic, practical, down to earth. The loss of illusions is thus a desirable and normal result of maturity. . . .

"The process of losing or reducing illusions involves diverse feelings—disappointment, joy, relief, bitterness, grief, wonder, freedom—and has diverse outcomes. A man may feel bereft and have the experience of suffering an irreparable loss. He may also feel liberated [and] free to develop more flexible values. . . ."[9]

For smokers, an important part of this deep look into one's past life frequently includes a growing understanding of the central role smoking has played as one of the key defenses in his or her personality structure. Smokers going through this kind of self-analysis may feel both the thrill of increased understanding and intense anxiety at the imagined loss of control they might experience if their smoking habit were to come to an end. It is most important, at this stage, that smokers find someone with whom they can discuss these feelings.

A spouse, a support person, a friend or "buddy" going through the same process, a support group composed of other smokers who are examining the role smoking plays in their own lives, or a sympathetic former smoker—all can be particularly helpful in calming a smoker's fears through sharing of fantasies. The friend, group, or buddy provides a supportive environment in which prospective quitters can let go of some of their own strict controls, can let themselves express their feelings more directly, and can allow some temporary loss of control to occur.

The Helper-Benefit Principle

Another benefit of making use of a friend, buddy, or group during this period of taking stock is that you can increase your chances of success in modifying your own smoking behavior by helping someone else do so at the same time. You will increase your chances of successful quitting if you provide support to another potential quitter. And by helping others quit after you become an ex-smoker, you can cut your chances of relapsing. Studies show that as an additional reward, such helpers experience significant positive changes in self-image.[10]

Quitting and Self-Analysis

The prospective quitter usually comes to realize that he or she is using smoking as an attempt to deal with anxiety, as a means of coping with unacceptable drives and urges, or as an expression of rebelliousness and defiance of authority. The process of preparing to quit provides a time in which these matters can be opened up, permitting the smoker to seek some resolution of these issues.[11]

The principal task, during the period leading up to and following quitting, is to become fully conscious of the way the addictive cycle plays itself out in one's life. In general outline, it works something like this:

- The smoker is faced with one or more undesirable aspects of reality.

- The smoker stops coping and lights a cigarette. Instead of working to resolve the situation, he or she chooses to seek refuge in a familiar practice that has pleasant effects.

- The more frequently this cycle occurs, the less capable the smoker feels of dealing with the anxieties and uncertainties that triggered the urge to smoke in the first place.

- Life is now increasingly viewed as a burden, a succession of unpleasant and useless struggles. Smoking is seen as a way to survive. Efforts to quit are viewed as meeting with inevitable failure.

- Eventually the cigarette comes to serve as a permanent psychological crutch the smoker cannot imagine doing without.[12]

How does one break this vicious cycle?

- The smoker finally realizes that it is smoking that has become the principal problem.

- Rather than seeming to be a positive aspect of one's life, smoking now increasingly is experienced as a noxious and unpleasant burden.

- The prospective quitter realizes that it is possible to take steps to build up his readiness to quit by means of requests for social support, adopting a healthier lifestyle, managing stress more effectively, making other positive life decisions, and becoming more aware of the role smoking plays in his life.

- The smoker experiences a number of small successes that show him he can take more control over his smoking: He cuts down on his number of cigarettes per day, he changes brands, he goes for longer and longer periods without smoking.

- When he finally feels that he is ready, he stops smoking altogether. While he may or may not experience a few additional slips, he eventually succeeds.

Through this long and complex process, the driving force is a strong and healthy urge on the smoker's part to transform the young adult self into a mature adult self wiser and more aware than before. This new, mature self is more experienced, less subject to illusions, less ego-centered, and more conscious of an urge to do good for others. Trading in one's younger illusions for a more realistic knowledge of limitations and potentials is an essential step toward taking a more complete kind of responsibility for one's actions, and a way to begin building a positive legacy in the world.[13]

Quitting and Grieving

Many smokers who quit go through a process that includes a large element of grieving. As one smoker said: "It wasn't until I was into my fourth week that I suddenly realized that I was experiencing a grief reaction association with the loss of a special friend—my cigarette! Once I understood the theoretical basis for my behavior, I was able to accept it and to begin developing coping strategies. Having experienced a previous loss through divorce, I again mustered up the energy and the determination to deal with my feelings of grief and loss. One of the strategies I used was to share my feelings of loss with my family and with Ann, who became my primary support person."

The experience of grief was mentioned by many of the successful quitters we spoke with. For many smokers, cigarettes represent one of the few constant and reliable sources of support in their lives. While some smokers are able to make the transition to nonsmoking with relative ease, some—especially those who are heavily addicted—may require several months to successfully mourn the loss of an important companion and to learn to reinvest their emotional capital in new and more productive areas. As Christen and Cooper write: "The depth of psychological grief and emptiness experienced by an individual after quitting can be remarkable. At one of our clinics, a woman was overheard to say that she mourned more when she quit smoking than she did when her husband died."[14]

Elaine Richard and Ann C. Shepard describe the process of quitting in terms of some of the stages of grief Elisabeth Kübler-Ross observed in seriously ill and dying patients:

- Denial—The smoker denies the health risks of smoking. For example, one might rationalize: "It won't happen to me. I won't get lung cancer or heart disease. I'll be one of the lucky ones. I'm an exception to the rule."

- Anger—Once the smoker quits, he or she is subject to angry outbursts and tends to overreact to both people and situations. Such anger is directed both at smokers who continue to smoke and at nonsmokers who do not appreciate the magnitude of the effort the quitter is making.

- Depression—The period of psychological withdrawal may include feelings of profound loss or grief, an experience of emptiness or lack of meaning. This feeling has been described by a wide variety of smokers as "like losing a good friend."

- Acceptance—Although it may take several weeks or months for them to do so, successful quitters finally arrive at a peaceful and, in many cases, enthusiastic acceptance of this major change in their lives. In many cases, this acceptance process can be speeded up by identifying and expressing any and all feelings experienced both before and after quitting.[15]

The "Final Straw"

Caroline is a forty-two-old San Francisco journalist who had quit smoking six months before this interview.

"I worked up to quitting for a year or more before I finally smoked my last cigarette," she recalls. "I was becoming more and more irritated with my smoking. And as a single woman in my early forties, I could no longer pretend that smoking was a glamorous addition to my life. When I went to parties, it was a growing embarrassment to find myself out on the back porch with the one or two other smokers—or sometimes totally alone.

"I spent several months just looking at the way I used cigarettes. I became convinced that I was using them to make up for the insane demands of my job, and for my almost total lack of a social life. I desperately needed to make new friends, and to see my existing friends more often. Yet my smoking was preventing me from doing that.

"The final straw was the way my smoking affected my running. Don't laugh—I was a regular runner for several years before I quit. Running had become a regular part of my life, but I just couldn't extend my range beyond 2 or 3 miles.

"I'd thought about it and thought about it. I'd managed to cut down to about 20 cigarettes a day. At last the day came when I was finally ready to quit. And I was absolutely sure I could do it.

"About that time I was invited to spend the weekend with some friends up in Oregon. Several of them were smokers. I knew that wouldn't be a good time to quit, but I resolved that I would do so as soon as the weekend was over. I had my last cigarette before I got on the plane to come home. For the first time in my life, I asked for a seat in the nonsmoking section. When I got home I treated myself to a succession of long, hot baths.

"My physical withdrawal symptoms were surprisingly mild. The psychological symptoms were somewhat more troublesome. All kinds of things seemed to go wrong during the month after I quit. For a few days there, it really *did* feel as if the universe was conspiring to give me an excuse to start smoking again. But I never really had any serious doubts about succeeding.

"After I quit, I found I had a lot of extra energy to get rid of. It was a wonderful excuse to call up friends and ask them to go somewhere with me, to help me to get through those first difficult days. Nobody turned me down. Everyone seemed delighted that I'd become a nonsmoker at last.

"I think the key to my success was the fact that I didn't push myself. I waited until I was really ready. My desire to quit had been building and building to the point where it was finally very easy for me to say, 'All right, no more. This is my last cigarette.'

"Since I quit I've gradually increased my running to 5 miles a day. And I'm feeling better than I have in years."

Tips from Successful Ex-Smokers

"I quit cigarettes at a very difficult time in my life. It took me a long time to 'hit bottom,' but when I did, I hit hard. Deep in my guts I finally got it: These cigarettes were not *good* for me.

"It was like I'd reached the bottom of a deep, dark well. I was really stuck. It was a time of great conflict in my life. And then, somehow, I found within it a place of great quiet and great resolve. I was going to survive. The only way I had to go was up.

"At that point it really helps if you can let down your normal defenses enough to reach out to others. This is the time you really need support. You find out who your *real* friends truly are.

"I decided I was going to make a number of major changes and really take control of my life. Quitting smoking was just one part of the package. I needed to turn all this seeming disaster and misfortune around and get my life going in a good direction. With a lot of work and a lot of help, I was able to do exactly that. I feel 200 times better about myself for having the determination and perseverance to quit."

● ● ●

"Once you make it through the quitting process, you're suddenly a tremendous resource for others who *haven't* yet been able to quit. This does *not* mean that you should begin bugging your smoking friends unmercifully. Just indicate your willingness to be of help if they should ever decide to quit. You may be surprised at the response."

● ● ●

"When I started looking at the things that were keeping me from quitting, I discovered that a very important one was the fact that my father had been a smoker all his life. I had a difficult and tangled relationship with my father. He died of a heart attack seven years ago. His smoking probably caused it. It seems weird to say this, but I realized that part of me felt that, in quitting, I would be betraying my father.

"That really freaked me out. I spent several sessions discussing it with a psychologist. He had me role-play a scene in which I asked my father to forgive me for all the things I'd done that hurt him. Then I role-played my father, asking *me* to forgive *him*.

"I finally asked him how he felt about my quitting. He said that with all the things we know now, I'd be an idiot not to. He said that if he'd known then what we know now, he might still be alive.

"I'm not sure whether that was the reason or not, but I did succeed in quitting right after that."

• • •

"I think the key to quitting is to allow yourself to fully acknowledge the pain. Smokers use smoking to anesthetize unwelcome or unpleasant feelings. We smoke because we're afraid of feeling things. But we block out our feeling at the expense of some of the best parts of our lives.

"My best advice for new quitters is to let it all out in whatever form seems most comfortable. If you're feeling lonely and scared, call up a friend. Ask your wife or husband for a hug. Talk it out, write it out, draw a picture or write a song about it, but you've got to let yourself feel it all—the joy and the pain both—without denying anything."

• • •

"The hardest part of dealing with withdrawal is the crazy urge to want to take a pill or wave a magic wand

and just make it all go away, poof. Smoking is about control, and it's the feeling of being out of control that's so hard to handle, not the actual symptoms.''

* * *

"I think the key is focusing on the positive. Build up the good things in your life, and the smoking will go away by itself. The thing I did that helped me the most was to set up one really fun thing to do every single day."

Characteristics of Successful Quitters

The available evidence suggests that these successful ex-smokers' suggestions about opening yourself to feelings and being open to learning new things about yourself are precisely on target. Those who succeed in quitting are much more likely than unsuccessful quitters to come to some important realizations about themselves. Successful quitters are typically highly dissatisfied with themselves for their smoking, perceive themselves as being overly dependent on cigarettes, and see themselves as more negatively affected by their habit. They are more flexible and more strongly determined to quit. They make more efforts to minimize the obstacles to quitting. They are more willing to tolerate discomfort, but in fact have an easier time going through withdrawal than the unsuccessful quitters.[16]

Quitting as Opportunity

In the process of quitting, a great deal of energy and attention is released, and is thus available to be placed elsewhere. Prospective quitters should plan in advance where they wish to invest it—in friends, family, a regular exercise program, a new project, or meditative practices that will bring a new peacefulness to their lives.

The period before, during, and after quitting is an opportunity to allow yourself to become more aware, more relaxed, and more accepting of the way you really are and the way the world really is. It provides a chance to let go of some of your old habits of self-protective control. It is a unique opportunity to be open to new life, to assume full power as a responsible adult and, in so doing, to allow yourself to live more fully.

As one successful ex-smoker explained: "Sure there were some tough times. It was a hard two or three months. There was a lot of anguish and a deep sense of loss. But there was a lot of richness and excitement, too, a lot of laughter, and a tremendous feeling of rightness and relief. There was an amazing sense of being reborn, of being given a second chance.

"I knew I was going to make it. Because even at the hardest times, I never doubted that the whole thing was going to be a totally positive experience. The pain I was feeling was just the old, deadened parts of myself coming back to life again."

How to Send a Copy of *The No-Nag, No-Guilt, Do-It-Your-Own-Way Guide to Quitting Smoking* to a Friend

Every single one of our advance readers told us they'd like to send a copy of *The No-Nag, No-Guilt, Do-It-Your-Own-Way Guide to Quitting Smoking* to one or more friends. They suggested that many of our readers might feel the same way.

Can you think of friends or family members *you* would like to send a copy to? If so, we'd be delighted to do all the work for you, and to enclose any card or message you'd like to send along. (Dr. Ferguson will be glad to autograph copies on request.) Or you may prefer to have extra copies sent directly to you, to give or loan to friends as you choose.

Please enclose $4.95 per book plus $2.00 postage and handling for each address (regardless of the number of books ordered). Be sure to provide the name and complete address (including zip code) of each recipient. And please enclose your *own* address and a daytime phone number, in case we have any questions. Send orders to:

Center for Self-Care Studies
3805 Stevenson Avenue
Austin TX 78703
(512) 472-1333

You can bill your purchase to your VISA or MasterCard. Please tell us which card you are using and include the exact name on the card, the card number, the expiration date, and your signature. Discounts available on purchases of six or more books shipped to a single address. Please write for details.

(You may also want to consider sending a friend our audio tape program based on *The No-Nag, No-Guilt, Do-It-Your-Own-Way Guide to Quitting Smoking*—see p. 207.)

About *Helping Smokers Get Ready to Quit: A New Approach to the Toughest Problem in Health Promotion*

This professional manual, compiled by Dr. Ferguson in response to many requests from health professionals and employers, will be of special interst to:

- Health professionals and health educators who work with smokers.
- Those who run wellness or smoking cessation programs.
- Executives responsible for workplace smoking policies.

Helping Smokers Get Ready to Quit provides the health professional and employer with a detailed overview of self-help approaches which can be used to *empower* rather than *embarrass* the smoker and induce guilt and shame. While most conventional approaches to smoking cessation see the smoker as the *problem* and assume that the only way to 'cure' smoking is to run the smoker through a professionally directed program, this guilt-free approach seeks to make the smoker (and his or her co-workers, immediate friends, and family members) into a primary *resource* for choosing and pursuing positive health options.

Ths new approach was suggested by American Cancer Society studies, which show that more than 90 percent of successful quitters discontinue their habit without attending a formal smoking cessation program, and by Dr. Ferguson's research for *The No-Nag, No-Guilt, Do-It-Your-Own-Way Guide to Quitting Smoking*, which revealed that smokers want a great deal more wellness information than traditional smoking cessation programs normally provide. The smokers in Dr. Ferguson's study emphasized the fact that they wanted this information presented in a nonjudgmental, nonauthoritarian way that *supports*, rather than *undermines*, thcir sense of themselves as capable, competent people.

Helping Smokers Get Ready to Quit includes a detailed curriculum for a new type of educational event for health-concerned smokers. This revolutionary two-and-a-half-hour workshop was developed by Dr. Ferguson for the Seton Hospital Good Health School in Austin, Texas.

Helping Smokers Get Ready to Quit also includes:

- A model grant proposal for funding your own program based on these principles.
- Guidelines for developing a workplace policy on smoking.
- An annotated bibliography of key smoking cessation resources.

Moneyback guarantee: Return within 30 days if not 100 percent satisfied.

Those who order the manual will automatically receive announcements of future publications and will be informed of Dr. Ferguson's presentations and workshops in their home region.

Wellness for Smokers: A New Approach to the Toughest Problem in Health Promotion is available for $34.95 (plus $2.00 postage and handling) from The Center for Self-Care Studies, 3805 Stevenson Avenue, Austin TX 78703, (512) 472-1333 VISA/MasterCard accepted. Quantity discounts available. Institutions may request to be billed.

APPENDIX I
How to Help a Health-Concerned Smoker

~~~~~~~~~~~~~~~~~~~~~~~~~~~~~~~

To judge from the comments of the smokers we interviewed, *most nonsmokers simply do not know how best to help a health-concerned smoker*. The smokers we interviewed told us they received little support or encouragement from their nonsmoking friends. Most of the things their nonsmoking friends said ranged from minor nagging to shockingly rude put-downs.

We could only conclude that most nonsmokers with smoking friends are missing an important opportunity. Nonsmoking friends *can* play a major role in helping a health-concerned smoker cut down or quit, but to do so most effectively, they should reinforce the idea that it is possible for smokers to take control of their smoking, while remaining supportive of the smoker as a person. The ideal approach does *not* include hostile confrontation, threats, put-downs, preaching, or nagging. As Cristen and Cooper write, ''Coercive, scare-type approaches or those based on excessive judgment, rationality, and criticism have little place in a quit-smoking program. 'Hard-sell' approaches, which attempt to induce guilt or shame in smokers, should be avoided because they may overwhelm the ego rather than inform, assist, or strengthen it. These approaches leave the smoker afraid, ashamed, or guilt-ridden, and he may reach for another cigarette to soothe these painful feelings."[1]

The smokers we interviewed suggested the following guidelines for concerned nonsmokers who wish to support a friend or family member's efforts to reduce their health risk:

- Separate the smoker from the smoking. Let the person know that you will continue to care about them no matter *what* they decide to do about their smoking.

- Try to envision the problem from the smoker's point of view. Smoking can help you deal with stress. It can help you relax. It can help you concentrate. It can keep you from becoming bored. It can be such a cherished part of your life pattern that giving it up would be like losing a good friend.

- Smoking is a powerful physical and psychological addiction. Quitting can be painfully difficult. Thus, the temptation to simply ignore the negative health effects of smoking can be very strong. Smokers who do exhibit the courage to confront this dilemma deserve compassion and understanding, not ridicule and blame. A supportive relationship with a caring and understanding nonsmoking friend can make the smoker feel more secure and can thus help provide the positive psychological motivation for change.

- Don't tell your smoking friends what to do. Encourage them to do what *they* think is best. Remember, it is only when *they* want to do something about their smoking that progress can occur.

- Encourage your smoking friends to engage in healthful, enjoyable activities that are incompatible with smoking (walking, hiking, volleyball, swimming, tennis, etc.) and activities at which smoking is not allowed (religious services, concerts, etc.).

- It is perfectly all right to ask your smoking friends not to smoke in your presence or in your house or car, but you should do so in a courteous, nonjudgmental way.

Refraining from open criticism does not mean that you cannot subtly "train" your smoking friends to follow more healthful practices.

Karen Pryor, animal trainer and author of *Don't Shoot the Dog: The New Art of Teaching and Training*, offers the following guidelines:

"The key to training a friend to cut down or quit is to totally ignore all the bothersome or offensive aspects of their smoking behavior, while giving positive reinforcement for periods of nonsmoking," says Pryor. "You must attempt to reinforce the *absence* of the undesired behavior. In the beginning, smokers may go only ten or fifteen minutes at a time without smoking," Pryor explains. "But if you lavish them with praise and attention during these nonsmoking periods, you'll find that they'll go longer and longer without a cigarette.

"You don't even have to *mention* the smoking," Pryor says. "Just shower them with hugs and kisses, give them your full attention, laugh at their jokes, or whatever's appropriate. This method will work whether they realize what you're doing or not. The key thing to remember is that you must never, never get into an open confrontation, because if the smoker feels abused or mistreated, he or she will simply get back at you by smoking even more."[2] Pryor's excellent book provides additional tips on training the behavior of friends and family members in positive directions.[3]

While you should, at all costs, avoid nagging your friends and family members about their smoking, there *is* a role for supportive, loving confrontation. However, such confrontation should be used very sparingly. The approach used by one of the successful quitters we interviewed can serve as a good example of the *right* way to go about it.

Frank is a forty-one-year-old lawyer. He has been a nonsmoker for four years. His mother, who is currently sixty-eight, had, until recently, smoked all her adult life.

"Although I'd quit myself, I had never been a crusader about getting others to do so," Frank remembers. "I'd certainly never said anything about my mother's smoking. But the time finally came when my brothers and sisters and I all had to accept the fact that Mom's health wasn't as good as it had been. She was becoming increasingly short of breath, and would need to stop and rest frequently. Her annual physical examination showed that her cholesterol level was dangerously high. Yet she was still smoking like a chimney.

"Thanksgiving was coming up and as usual we were planning a big family gathering. I told my other brothers and sisters I was going to take Mom aside and tell her how worried I'd become about her smoking. Most of them decided that they would do likewise. We all ended up telling her how much we loved her and how terrible we would all feel if anything were to happen. She wrote to us all the next week to tell us how much our expressions of concern had meant to her. And she said that she was going to work on the problem. On the first of January she quit for good."

Love and understanding from friends and family are particularly important in the days and weeks immediately after quitting. Here are some guidelines for supporting a friend during this difficult time:

- Let your friend know that you are overjoyed that he is quitting and that you are confident he will be able to remain smoke-free.

- Make a commitment to "adopt" the recent quitter. Tell your friend that during this quitting period, you will be delighted to provide whatever support you can. This should include encouragement as well as such mundane services as preparing food, cleaning house, taking care of the children, doing the laundry.

- Make yourself available as frequently as possible, either in person or by phone, for your adoptee's first few days as a nonsmoker. Be prepared to listen to his hostile or angry feelings. Accept the fact that he may react to the stresses of withdrawal by lashing out verbally at whoever is around—you included. Be prepared for somewhat bizarre behavior. Accept the fact that the loss of his cherished habit may be very painful to him. Be prepared to forgive him in advance, and encourage him to do anything he needs to do to get through this difficult time. Smoking is a habit that takes a long time to learn; it can take a long time to unlearn.

- After the first few days, the worst should be over. Arrange to see your friend regularly for several weeks thereafter, and to check in with him regularly for the remainder of his first year as a nonsmoker.

- Help your friend keep as far away from smokers and from cigarettes as possible. It is worth considerable trouble and inconvenience to avoid a situation in which it could be all too easy for your friend to decide to smoke "just one cigarette."

- Consider giving up something yourself—candy, desserts, or coffee—for the first days or weeks of your adoptee's new life as a nonsmoker to show that you really care.

- Encourage your friend to talk about what he is feeling or experiencing. Listen sympathetically and supportively, without judging or offering advice.

- Send flowers or take your adoptee to dinner (to a restaurant with a no-smoking section) to celebrate his first week or first month as a nonsmoker.

- Offer direct rewards for continued nonsmoking— (I'll give you $50 if you can go without smoking for 100 days'').

- Offer indirect rewards (''I'll give each of your kids $50 if you can go without smoking for 100 days'').

If you are a smoker, be aware that you may feel threatened by a friend's efforts to quit. Knowing that your friend desperately wants to quit may make you painfully aware of the ways smoking is harming your *own* body. You may justifiably feel that if she is successful in quitting, she will now begin to avoid you because you are a smoker. Share these concerns with your friend. Make a deal with your friend: You will support the way she has chosen to deal with smoking if she will support the way you have chosen to deal with it.

Realize that to succeed in the decision she has made, she is in great need of your support. Here are some of the things you can do to help:

- The smell of smoke can be extremely tempting to a recent quitter, particularly during the first few days after quitting. Make a commitment to your friend that you will not smoke in her presence until she invites you to do so.

- Your friend may go through a period of being irritable and grumpy in the weeks or months immediately after quitting. She will greatly appreciate it if you are understanding and accepting of this short-lived irritability and refrain from suggestions that a cigarette might calm her nerves.

- Be aware that as a quitter becomes a successful nonsmoker, she may become more critical of smokers, cigarette ads, tobacco companies, and everything else associated with her former habit. If this occurs, remind her of your "deal," and gently explain that she is exhibiting some of the warning signs of becoming a self-righteous ex-smoker.

- Smoking together can be an important part of a friendship. Show your friend you really care for her by working with her to develop other activities that you can now do together.

- If you are supportive and understanding during your friend's efforts to become a nonsmoker, then you can be sure that if and when you decide to cut down or quit, you will be able to count on her encouragement, support, and understanding during this difficult time in *your* life.

APPENDIX II
Medical Tests Affected
by Smoking

Results of the tests listed below can be affected by smoking. If you smoke and are planning to have any of these tests, be sure your health professional is aware of your present smoking level.

Test	How Influenced by Smoking	Significance
Carbon Monoxide Blood Levels	Increased	Carbon monoxide binds to the hemoglobin in red blood cells, converting it into a form incapable of carrying oxygen to the body. High blood levels make a smoker's heart work harder.
Red Blood Cell Count	Increased	Probably due to the carbon monoxide in tobacco smoke. Returns to normal within a few weeks of quitting.

Test	How Influenced by Smoking	Significance
White Blood Cell Count	Increased	Increased WBC may be interpreted as evidence of infection.
Hematocrit	Increased	Probably due to the carbon monoxide in tobacco smoke. Returns to normal within a few weeks of quitting.
Hemoglobin	Increased	Probably due to the carbon monoxide in tobacco smoke. Returns to normal within a few weeks of quitting.
Clotting Tests	The blood of healthy smokers clots faster than that of nonsmokers.	Decreased clotting time may be mistaken for clotting disorder.
High-density Lipoprotein Levels (HDL)	Decreased	May increase risk of heart disease. (HDL has a protective effect.) Returns to normal within a year of quitting.
Bilirubin Blood Levels	Decreased	Decreased values on this test may be interpreted as evidence of hepatitis, cirrhosis, mononucleosis, or gallstones.
CEA Antigens	Healthy smokers can have high blood levels of CEA antigens.	High CEA levels may be interpreted as evidence of cancer.

Test	How Influenced by Smoking	Significance
Alkaline Phosphatase Blood Levels	Increased	Increased values on this test may be interpreted as evidence of hepatitis, cirrhosis, blocked bile duct, bone tumors, or parathyroid deficiency.
SGOT (Serum Glutamic Oxalacetic Acid) Blood Levels	Decreased	No common diseases are associated with low SGOT levels.
Serum Protein Blood Levels	Decreased	Decreased values on this test may be interpreted as evidence of kidney disease, diabetes, congestive heart failure, or impaired absorption of food from the intestine.
Lung Function Tests	Lung function is impaired in many long-term smokers.	Smokers with impaired lung function are at increased risk of emphysema. Smokers over thirty-five should have their lung function measured at least every five years.
Upper GI Series	Smoking interferes with test results—probably by stimulating secretions in the stomach.	You will be asked to abstain from smoking for 12 hours before the test.

Test	How Influenced by Smoking	Significance
Electroencephalogram (EEG)	Alpha frequency brainwaves are decreased in smokers deprived of cigarettes.	Ask your clinician for guidelines for smoking for the 24 hours before the test.
Saliva thiocyanite	Positive only in smokers.	Used by some employers and insurance companies to verify nonsmoking status.

APPENDIX III
Drugs Affected by Smoking

The effects of the following drugs can be altered by smoking. If you smoke and are taking (or plan to take) any of these drugs, be sure to let your health professional know about your present smoking level and ask if you should modify the amount of the drug you are taking.

Drug	How Used	How Influenced by Smoking	Significance
Acetaminophen (Tylenol, Anacin-3, etc.)	Pain relief	Decreases blood levels.	Smokers may require higher doses.
Amobarbital (Amytal)	Sedative	Eliminated more quickly in smokers.	Smokers may require larger doses.
Benzodiazepines (Valium, Librium, Tranxene, Centrax, Halcion, Xanax)	Sleeping pills, sedatives	Drugs are eliminated more rapidly by smokers.	Smokers may need higher doses.

Drug	How Used	How Influenced by Smoking	Significance
Caffeine	Stimulant	Caffeine is eliminated more rapidly by smokers.	Smokers experience less stimulation from caffeine than nonsmokers.
Cimetidine (Tagamet)	Reduces production of acid in the stomach.	Blocks drug action.	Smokers should take medication at bedtime and should not smoke thereafter.
Furosemide	Diuretic (increases urine output)	Less effective in smokers.	Discuss with your physician.
Glutethimide (Doriden, etc.)	Sedative	Smoking enhances drug effects.	Smokers may need smaller doses.
Heparin	Anticlotting drug	Eliminated more rapidly in smokers.	Smokers may require larger doses.
Oral Contraceptives	Birth control	Risk of clots, strokes, and heart attack increase—especially after age thirty-five and with more than 15 cigarettes per day.	Women over thirty-five who smoke should not use birth control pills.

Drug	How Used	How Influenced by Smoking	Significance
Pentazocine (Talwin)	Pain relief	Drug is excreted more quickly in smokers.	Increased maintenance doses may be needed.
Phenothiazines (Thorazine, Mellaril)	Tranquilizer	Decreased effect has been reported in smokers.	Discuss with your physician.
Phenylbutazine (Azolid, Butazolidin)	Antiarthritis drug	Drug is broken down more quickly in smokers.	Smokers may need higher doses.
Propoxyphene (Darvon, SK-65)	Pain relief	Reported less effective in smokers.	Discuss with your physician.
Postmenopausal estrogens (Premarin)	Postmenopausal hormone therapy	Estrogen is broken down more rapidly in smokers.	Discuss with your physician.
Propanolol (Inderal)	Heart problems, high blood pressure, migraines.	Reported less effective in smokers.	Discuss with your physician.
Theophylline	Asthma	Broken down more quickly in smokers.	Higher doses may be required.
Tricyclic antidepressants (Tofranil)	Antidepressant drug	Eliminated more quickly in smokers.	Smokers may require larger doses.

Drug	How Used	How Influenced by Smoking	Significance
Vitamin B$_{12}$ (Cyanocobalamin)	Vitamin used to treat B$_{12}$ deficiency	B$_{12}$ levels are decreased.	Smokers should be sure they have ample B$_{12}$ intake.
Vitamin C	Essential vitamin	Eliminated more rapidly in smokers.	Smokers should be sure they have ample Vitamin C intake.

APPENDIX IV
Tar, Nicotine, and Carbon Monoxide Content of U.S. Cigarettes

The values listed below were obtained when each brand was smoked by a smoking machine. The actual amounts of tar, nicotine, and carbon monoxide that reach a smoker's lungs can vary greatly from smoker to smoker, depending on the way the cigarette is smoked. Smokers can decrease their exposure to the harmful substances by smoking fewer cigarettes, taking fewer puffs per cigarette, taking smaller puffs, and by inhaling less or not at all. (Additional guidelines for choosing a low-tar cigarette and smoking it in a way that will reduce your exposure to the harmful substances in tobacco smoke are provided in chapter 7.)

Brand	Tar	Nicotine	CO
Cambridge Hard Pack			
Carlton			
Carlton 100			
Now			
Now 100		0.1	
Benson & Hedges	1	0.1	2

Brand	Tar	Nicotine	CO
Cambridge Soft Pack	1	0.1	1
Carlton 2 Soft Pack	1	0.1	1
Carlton Menthol	1	0.1	1
Carlton 100 Hard Pack	1	0.1	
Now	1	0.1	2
Now Menthol	1	0.1	1
Kool Ultra	2	0.1	1
Now 100 Menthol	2	0.2	1
Kent III	3	0.3	2
Now 100	3	0.3	2
Triumph	3	0.3	3
Triumph Menthol	3	0.3	2
Doral II	4	0.4	3
Doral II Menthol	4	0.4	3
Iceberg 100	4	0.3	4
Kent III 100	4	0.4	5
Kool Ultra 100	4	0.4	3
Merit Ultra Lites 100	4	0.4	4
Tareyton Lights	4	0.4	4
Triumph 100	4	0.4	5
Triumph 100 Menthol	4	0.4	4
Benson & Hedges Ultra Light	5	0.4	5
Benson & Hedges Ultra Light Menthol	5	0.4	5
Cambridge 100	5	0.4	5
Carlton 100	5	0.4	6
Carlton 100 Menthol	5	0.4	6
Merit Ultra Lights	5	0.4	5
Merit Ultra Lights Menthol	5	0.4	5
Merit Ultra Lights 100	5	0.4	6
Salem Ultra Menthol	5	0.4	6
Salem Ultra 100 Menthol	5	0.4	6
True	5	0.4	4

Brand	Tar	Nicotine	CO
True Menthol	5	0.4	5
Vantage Ultra Lights	5	0.4	6
Vantage Ultra Lights Menthol	5	0.4	6
Vantage Ultra Lights 100	5	0.5	6
Vantage Ultra Lights 100 Menthol	5	0.4	7
Winston Ultra Lights	5	0.4	6
Winston Ultra Lights 100	5	0.5	7
Bright Menthol	6	0.5	7
Bright 100 Menthol	6	0.5	7
Carlton 120	7	0.6	5
Carlton 120 Menthol	7	0.6	5
Pall Mall Extra Light	7	0.6	7
Tareyton Long Lights 100	7	0.6	7
True 100 Menthol	7	0.6	8
Belair 100 Menthol	8	0.6	7
Camel Lights	8	0.7	10
Kent Golden Lights Menthol	8	0.7	8
Kool Lights Menthol	8	0.7	9
L & M Lights	8	0.7	7
L & M Lights 100	8	0.8	6
Merit	8	0.5	9
Merit Menthol	8	0.5	10
More Lights 100	8	0.6	8
More Lights 100 Menthol	8	0.6	8
Newport Lights Menthol	8	0.7	8
Salem Slim Lights Menthol	8	0.7	9
True 100	8	0.6	8
Virginia Slims Lights 100	8	0.6	7
Virginia Slims Lights 100 Menthol	8	0.6	8
Winston Lights	8	0.7	9
Camel Lights	9	0.7	8

Brand	Tar	Nicotine	CO
Century Lights	9	0.7	11
Kent Golden Lights	9	0.8	9
Kent Golden Lights 100	9	0.8	10
Kent Golden Lights 100 Menthol	9	0.8	9
Kool Lights 100 Menthol	9	0.7	9
Merit 100 Menthol	9	0.7	11
Newport Lights Menthol	9	0.7	9
Old Gold Lights	9	0.8	10
Pall Mall Lights 100	9	0.7	9
Parliament Lights	9	0.6	9
Raleigh Lights 100	9	0.7	9
Salem Lights Menthol	9	0.7	11
Salem Lights 100 Menthol	9	0.7	11
Satin 100 Menthol	9	0.8	10
Vantage Menthol	9	0.7	12
Vantage 100	9	0.7	11
Vantage 100 Menthol	9	0.7	11
Belair Menthol	10	0.7	9
Benson & Hedges Lights 100	10	0.7	11
Benson & Hedges Lights 100 Menthol	10	0.7	10
Kool Milds Menthol	10	0.7	11
Lucky Strike	10	0.8	10
Marlboro Lights	10	0.7	11
Marlboro Lights 100	10	0.7	11
Merit 100	10	0.7	12
Newport Lights 100 Menthol	10	0.8	10
Raleigh Lights	10	0.8	10
Satin 100	10	0.9	11
Vantage	10	0.7	12
Viceroy Rich Lights	10	0.7	10
Camel Lights 100	11	0.8	14
Kool Milds 100 Menthol	11	0.8	12

Brand	Tar	Nicotine	CO
Lucky Strike Hard Pack	11	0.8	10
Lucky Strike 100	11	0.9	10
Silva Thins	11	0.9	9
Silva Thins 100 Menthol	11	0.9	8
Viceroy Rich Lights 100	11	0.8	11
Winston Lights 100	11	0.8	13
Eve Lights 100	12	0.9	9
Eve Lights 100 Menthol	12	0.9	9
Kent Hard Pack	12	0.9	11
Kent Soft Pack	12	0.9	10
Multifilter	12	0.8	10
Multifilter Menthol	12	0.8	10
Newport Red	12	0.9	13
Pall Mall Light 100 Menthol	12	1.0	11
Parliament Lights 100	12	0.8	11
Players	12	0.8	11
Players Menthol	12	0.8	11
Dorado	13	0.9	12
Kent 100	13	1.0	11
L & M	13	0.9	13
Lark Lights	13	0.9	12
Lark Lights 100	13	1.0	13
Players 100	13	0.9	12
Tareyton	13	0.9	14
Tareyton 100	13	0.9	15
Century	14	0.9	16
Eve Lights 120	14	1.1	11
Eve Lights 120 Menthol	14	1.1	11
Galaxy	14	0.9	13
Kool Super Longs 100 Menthol	14	0.9	15
L & M 100	14	1.0	13
Lark	14	0.9	13
Newport Red	14	1.0	15

Brand	Tar	Nicotine	CO
Saratoga 120	14	0.9	13
Saratoga 120 Menthol	14	0.9	13
St. Moritz 100	14	1.1	13
St. Moritz 100 Menthol	14	1.1	13
Viceroy Super Long 100	14	0.9	16
Virginia Slims 100	14	0.9	12
Virginia Slims 100 Menthol	14	0.9	12
Benson & Hedges	15	1.1	11
Kent 100 Menthol	15	1.2	14
Lark 100	15	1.0	15
Montclair Menthol	15	1.0	15
Pall Mall 100	15	1.1	15
Raleigh	15	0.9	16
Richland Menthol	15	1.0	13
Alpine Menthol	16	0.9	14
Benson & Hedges 100	16	1.0	15
Benson & Hedges 100 Menthol	16	1.0	15
Camel Hard Pack	16	1.1	15
Camel Soft Pack	16	1.1	14
Kool Menthol Hard Pack	16	1.1	15
Kool Menthol Soft Pack	16	1.1	14
Marlboro	16	1.0	14
Marlboro	16	1.0	15
Marlboro Menthol	16	1.0	14
Marlboro 100 Hard Pack	16	1.0	14
Marlboro 100 Soft Pack	16	1.0	15
More 120 Menthol	16	1.2	19
Newport Menthol	16	1.1	15
Picayune	16	1.0	12
Raleigh 100	16	1.0	17
Richland	16	1.1	13
Salem Menthol	16	1.1	18
Salem 100 Menthol	16	1.2	15

Brand	Tar	Nicotine	CO
Viceroy	16	0.9	16
Winston Hard Pack	16	1.1	14
Winston Soft Pack	16	1.1	15
Winston International 100	16	1.1	14
More 120	17	1.2	20
Newport Menthol	17	1.2	17
Old Gold Filter	17	1.3	18
Pall Mall	17	1.1	16
Philip Morris International	17	1.1	16
Philip Morris International Menthol	17	1.1	16
Tall 120 Menthol	17	1.3	17
Winston 100	17	1.2	16
Half & Half	18	1.3	17
Max 120	18	1.4	17
Chesterfield	19	1.2	11
Max 120 Menthol	19	1.4	17
Newport 100 Menthol	19	1.5	20
Spring 100 Menthol	19	1.1	16
Kool Menthol	20	1.2	14
Old Gold Filter 100	20	1.5	20
Tall 120	20	1.5	19
Camel	21	1.4	13
Philip Morris	21	1.2	12
Chesterfield	22	1.5	13
English Ovals	23	1.8	11
Lucky Strike	23	1.4	16
Pall Mall	23	1.3	15
Herbert Tareyton	24	1.5	16
Players	25	1.9	15
Raleigh	25	1.4	16
Old Gold Straight	26	1.6	17
Philip Morris Commander	26	1.6	14
Bull Durham	28	1.8	23

Brand	Tar	Nicotine	CO
English Ovals	28	2.1	14

Tar—total particulate matter less nicotine and water in milligrams per cigarette.
Nicotine—total alkaloids in milligrams per cigarette.
Carbon Monoxide (CO)—in milligrams per cigarette.
*—Tar below 0.5 milligrams, nicotine below 0.05 milligrams, or carbon monoxide below 0.5 milligrams per cigarette.

Source : "Tar, Nicotine and Carbon Monoxide of the Smoke of 207 Varieties of Domestic Cigarettes." Federal Trade Commission Report, January 1985.

APPENDIX V
Smoker Survey Results

1. How have the attitudes of nonsmokers changed in the last five to ten years?

   Nonsmokers are now *much more*
   tolerant of smoking.   0%
   Nonsmokers are now *somewhat more*
   tolerant of smoking.   0%
   Nonsmokers' attitudes are pretty
   much unchanged.   3%
   Nonsmokers are now *somewhat less*
   tolerant of smoking.   17%
   Nonsmokers are now *much less*
   tolerant of smoking.   80%

2. Which of the following changes in nonsmokers' behavior have you noticed in the last few years?

Rank	Change	% Citing
1.	I'm now more likely to ask permission to smoke when visiting a nonsmoking friend.	91%

2. Friends and family members are now more likely to express concerns about my smoking. 79%

3. I am now more likely to refrain from smoking when nonsmokers are present. 75%

4. Nonsmokers in restaurants are now more likely to say that my smoking bothers them. 68%

5. I now feel guiltier about my smoking than I did a few years ago. 49%

3. Rate each of the following possible benefits of smoking on a scale of 1 to 10, with 10 being a very major benefit and 1 being no benefit.

Rank	Benefit	Score
1.	Helps me deal with stressful situations.	6.28
2.	Provides a pleasant and enjoyable break from work.	6.27
3.	Helps me unwind and relax.	6.15
4. (tie)	Helps me deal with painful or unpleasant situations.	4.92
4. (tie)	Prevents unpleasant withdrawal symptoms.	4.92
5.	Helps me deal with an overstimulating environment.	4.88
6.	I enjoy the physical sensation of lighting and handling a cigarette.	4.63
7.	Keeps me from feeling bored.	4.14
8.	Increases my enjoyment of pleasant experiences.	4.03
9.	Helps me feel comfortable in social situations.	3.77
10.	Helps me concentrate.	3.43

4. Rate each of the following possible drawbacks of smoking on a scale of 1 to 10, with 10 being a very major drawback and 1 being no drawback.

Rank	Drawback	Score
1.	I worry that it's bad for my health.	8.02
2.	Smoking makes my clothes, hair, home, and office smell bad.	6.35
3.	I get out of breath more easily because of my smoking.	6.15
4.	I spend too much money on cigarettes.	5.93
5.	I feel that other people disapprove of my smoking.	5.53
6.	I worry that smoking might be a health risk for others.	4.75
7.	I have more frequent colds, coughs, and sore throats.	4.13
8.	I feel that I am setting a bad example for others.	4.07
9.	Some people don't want to be my friend because I smoke.	2.20

5. Has smoking even been an issue in your romantic relationship(s)?

Never an issue	60%
A minor issue	28%
A major issue	12%

6. How guilty do you feel about the harm you may be doing to your own health by smoking?

Guilt level = 7.02 (On a scale of 1 to 10, with 10 representing extremely guilty.)

7. How guilty do you feel about the possibility that your smoking may encourage others to smoke?

   Guilt level = 3.54

8. How guilty do you feel about the possibility that your smoking may harm the health of friends and family?

   Guilt level = 4.10

9. Have you ever attempted to quit?

Have never wanted to quit	6%
Have wanted to quit but have never tried.	10%
Have tried, but have not succeeded.	24%
Have tried and succeeded, but started smoking again.	60%

10. What is the longest time you have gone without cigarettes since you started smoking?

Two days or more	85%
One week or more	76%
One year or more	28%

11. If you found a method that would make it possible for you to quit without experiencing the discomfort of withdrawal, would you be more likely to quit?

Would be more likely to quit.	84%
Would not be more likely to quit, minimal smoker, or not sure.	16%

12. Do you think you *will* quit smoking?

Will quit.	86%
No, minimal smoker, or not sure.	14%

13. If you continued smoking at *half* your present level, how many additional years of life would you gain?

    Average estimated gain among smokers
    who admit health risks.   6.52

14. If you quit today and never smoked again, how many additional years of life would you gain?

    Average estimated gain among smokers
    who admit health risks.   14.57

15. Would you like to take a greater measure of control of your smoking behavior?

    Yes   81%
    No   19% (half of these smoked less than 10 cigarettes per day)

16. Suppose there were a nonjudgmental, guilt-free guide for smokers that told you how to keep yourself healthier whether you decided to quit, cut down, or keep smoking. How useful would such a guide be to you in your efforts to take more control of your smoking?

    Extremely useful.   40%
    Moderately useful.   22%
    Somewhat useful.   29%
    Not at all useful.   9%

17. What topics should be covered in a resource guide for smokers? (On a scale of 1 to 10, 10 is extremely important, 1 is unimportant.)

Rank	*Topic*	*Score*
1.	How to *stay* a nonsmoker after you quit.	9.17
2.	The most effective ways of quitting.	8.88

3. The most effective ways of cutting down.   8.54

4. Getting ready to quit. What you need to know.   8.32

5. Do smokers have special needs for vitamins?   8.12

6. What smoking does to a smoker's body. 8.07

7. How to tell whether you're a high- or low-risk smoker.   7.97

8. Dealing with weight gain after you quit. 7.90

9. What withdrawal symptoms you may encounter if you quit.   7.85

10. How to cut your smoking risk through stress reduction.   7.80

11. Drugs, tools, and tips for the health-concerned smoker.   7.73

12. How to cut your smoking risks through exercise.   7.60

13. Tips from successful ex-smokers.   7.48

14. How smokers use smoking as a psychological tool.   7.46

15. How to cut your smoking risk by eating a healthier diet.   7.40

16. How to cut your risk by smoking less.   7.09

17. The case for controlled smoking.   6.65

18. Using nicotine gum to help you quit.   6.19

19. How to keep smoking from harming your family and friends.   6.04

20. The economic consequences of smoking.   4.88

21. How to get along with nonsmokers.   3.94

[Based on a survey of 100 adult smokers in San Francisco, California, and Austin, Texas. Subjects volunteered to be interviewed as part of a survey on the experiences and information needs of smokers. Subjects' ages ranged from twenty-two to sixty-five, though most were in their thirties and forties. Interviews were conducted by Tom Ferguson and Gail M. Schmidt between September 1985 and February 1986.]

NOTES

Chapter 1

1. The smokers in our study—like most of the readers of this book—were probably more aware of the negative health effects of smoking than the average smoker. See the description of our study in Appendix V.

2. "Americans Support Smoking Controls in Workplace, Agree that Smokers Should Refrain from Smoking Near Nonsmokers," *Smoking and Health Reporter*, Vol. 3, No. 2, p.4, January 1986. This poll was conducted in 1985 for the American Lung Association.

3. "Smoking Increasingly is Lower-Class Custom," *ASH Review*, September 1985, p.5.

4. This telephone survey of 1,253 American adults was conducted for Rodale Press by Louis Harris and Associates in November 1984. The results appear in *The Prevention Index '85: A Report Card on the Nation's Health*, Rodale Press, Emmaus, PA, 1985, pp. 6, 13.

5. Adapted from Patrick L. Remington et al. "Current Smoking Trends in the United States: The 1981-1983 Behavioral Risk Factors Surveys," *Journal of the American Medical Association*, Vol. 253, No. 20, pp. 2975-2978, May 24/31, 1985.

6. Anne S. Canfield, "How Not to Succeed in Business" (press release), Fleishman-Hillard Inc., Kansas City, MO, 1984.

7. William L. Weis, "Can You Afford to Hire Smokers?" *Personnel Administrator*, May 1981, pp. 71-78.

8. Leslie Goldberg, "Local Celebs Sound Off on Smoking," *San Francisco Examiner*, August 4, 1985, p. S-2.

9. Dedra Hauser, "In Tom Templin's War on Smokers, Revenge Isn't Sweet—It's Smelly," *Wall Street Journal*, September 20, 1983, p.29.

10. Stanley S. Scott, "Smokers Get a Raw Deal," *The New York Times*, December 29, 1984.

11. "American Doctors 'Refacing' Cigarette Billboards," *Smoking and Health Reporter*, Vol. 3, No. 4, p. 5, July 1986.

12. "No-Smoking Laws are Proliferating," *ASH Review*, July 1985, p.3.

13. "Effects of 'Passive Smoking' Lead Nonsmokers to Step Up Campaign" (excerpts), *Journal of the American Medical Association*, Vol. 253, No. 20, pp. 2937-2939, May 24/31, 1985. Excerpted in *Smoking and Health Review*, July 1985, p. 8.

14. This equation is adapted from a more general equation developed by Frank Riessman, Director of the National Self-Help Clearinghouse, New York, New York. Frank Riessman, personal communication, February 1986.

Chapter 2

1. M.A.H. Russell, "Realistic Goals for Smoking and Health: A Case for Safer Smoking," *Lancet*, Vol. 1, pp. 254-258, 1974.

2. Nina G. Schneider and Murray E. Jarvik, "Nicotine Gum vs. Placebo Gum: Comparisons of Withdrawal Symptoms and Success Rates," in *Pharmacological Adjuncts in Smoking Cessation*, NIDA Monograph Series #53, National Institute on Drug Abuse, Rockville, MD, 1985, p. 83.

3. Heather Ashton and Rob Stepney, "Smoking as a Psychological Tool," in Ashton and Stepney, *Smoking: Psychology and Pharmacology*, Tavistock Publications, London, 1982, pp. 91-119.

4. Lawrence M. Prescott, "Nasal Vasopressin Spray to Help Stop Smoking?" *Medical Tribune*, Vol. 25, No. 34, December 5, 1984; Sandra Blakeslee, "Smoking Depicted as an Addiction with Many Lures," *The New York Times*, December 25, 1984, pp. 33-34; William A. Check, "New Knowledge About Nicotine Effects," *Journal of the American Medical Association*, Vol. 247, pp. 2333, 2337-2338, May 7, 1982; Ovide F. Pomerleau and Cynthia S. Pomerleau, "Neuroregulators and the Reinforcement of Smoking: Towards a Bio-

behavioral Explanation," *Neuroscience and Biobehavioral Reviews*, Vol. 8, pp. 503-513, 1984.

5. Ovide F. Pomerleau and Cynthia S. Pomerleau, "Neuroregulators and the Reinforcement of Smoking Towards a Biobehavioral Explanation," *Neuroscience and Biobehavioral Reviews*, Vol 8. pp. 503-513, 1984.

6. Ashton and Stepney, pp. 91-119.

7. K. Wesnes and D.M. Warburton, "Smoking, Nicotine, and Human Performance," *Pharmacology and Therapeutics*, Vol. 21, pp. 189-208, 1978; Ashton and Stepney, p. 105.

8. Karin Andersson and G. Robert J. Hockey, "Effects of Cigarette Smoking on Memory," *Psychopharmacology*, Vol. 52, pp. 223-226, 1977.

9. K. Wesnes and D.M. Warburton, "The Effects of Cigarette Smoking and Nicotine Tablets Upon Human Attention," in R. E. Thornton (editor), *Smoking Behavior: Physiological and Psychological Influences*, Churchill Livingston, London, 1978, pp. 131-147.

10. Ashton and Stepney, p. 112.

11. Ibid.

12. W. L. Dunn, "Smoking as a Possible Inhibitor of Arousal," in K. Battig (editor), *Behavioral Effects of Nicotine*, S. Carger, Basel, 1978, pp. 20-21; Ashton and Stepney, p. 115.

13. J. M. Nelson, "Psychological Consequences of Chronic Nicotinisation: A Focus on Arousal," in Battig, *Behavioral Effects of Nicotine.*

14. G. H. Hall and C. F. Morrison, "New Evidence for a Relationship Between Tobacco Smoking, Nicotine Dependence, and Stress," *Nature*, Vol. 242, 1973, pp. 199-201.

15. N. W. Heimstra, "The Effects of Smoking on Mood Change," in W. L. Dunn (editor), *Smoking Behavior: Motives and Incentives*, Washington, Winston Publishers, 1973; R. R. Hutchinson and G. S. Emley, "Effects of Nicotine on Avoidance, Conditioned Suppression, and Aggression Response Measures in Animals and Man," in Dunn, *Smoking Behavior: Motives and Incentives.*

16. Olvide F. Pomerleau, Dennis C. Turk, and Joanne B. Fertig, "The Effects of Cigarette Smoking on Pain and Anxiety," *Addictive Behaviors*, Vol. 9, pp. 265-271, 1984.

17. Arden G. Christen and Kenneth H. Cooper, "Strategic Withdrawal from Cigarette Smoking," *CA: A Cancer Journal for Clinicians*, Vol. 29, No. 2, pp. 96-107, 1979.

18. The state of our present knowledge about the harmfulness of

nicotine is perhaps best summed up by pharmacologist Neal L. Benowitz: "Nicotine could play a role in the pathogenesis of many smoking-related diseases, although at present, there is no conclusive evidence it contributes to any." Benowitz's "Clinical Pharmacology of Nicotine," in *Annual Review of Medicine*, is in press.

Chapter 3

1. *The Health Consequences of Smoking: A Report of the Surgeon General: Cancer (1982), Cardiovascular Disease (1983), Chronic Obstructive Lung Disease (1984)*, Office of Smoking and Health, U.S. Department of Health and Human Services, Washington, D.C.

2. Bob Minzesheimer, "USA's Top Doc Gets Burned Up About Smoking," *USA Today*, December 20, 1985, p. 2A.

3. William Pollin, "The Role of the Addictive Process as a Key Step in the Causation of All Tobacco-Related Diseases," *The Journal of the American Medical Association*, Vol. 252, No. 20, November 23/30, 1984, p. 2874.

4. John D. Seffrin, "A Message from the Grave," *Smoking and Health Reporter*, Vol. 3, No. 3, p. 3, April 1986; John Urquhart and Klaus Heilmann, *Risk Watch—The Odds of Life*, Facts on File Publications, New York, 1984, pp. 85-90.

5. Personal communication, Victor J. Schoenback, University of North Carolina School of Public Health, Chapel Hill, June 1, 1986.

6. P. Bernfeld et al., "Subchronic Cigarette Smoke Inhalation Studies in Inbred Syrian Golden Hamsters That Develop Laryngeal Carcinoma Upon Chronic Exposure," *Journal of the National Cancer Institute*, Vol. 71, No. 3, pp. 619-623, September 1983.

7. Walter S. Ross, "What Happens When You Smoke," in *How to Stop Smoking Permanently*, Little, Brown, 1985, pp. 11-12.

8. Douglas Model, "Smoker's Face: An Underrated Clinical Sign?" *British Medical Journal*, Vol. 291, pp. 1760-1762, December 21/28, 1985.

9. "Carbon Monoxide Found in 80 percent of Cigarette Smokers," *The Wall Street Journal*, March 18, 1982, p. 33.

10. Personal communication, Dr. Irving Goldstein, Professor of Urology, New England Male Reproductive Center, Boston University Medical School, July 9, 1986.

11. "Tobacco Profoundly Affects Reproduction, Conference Report Shows," *Smoking and Health Reporter*, Vol. 3, No. 2, p. 3, January 1986.

12. Sonja McKinlay et al., "Smoking and Menopause in Women," *Annals of Internal Medicine*, Vol. 103, pp. 350-356; Donna Day Baird and Allen J. Wilcox, "Cigarette Smoking Associated with Delayed Conception," *Journal of the American Medical Association*, Vol. 253, No. 20, pp. 2979-2983, May 24/31, 1986; "Tobacco Profoundly Affects Reproduction, Conference Report Shows," *Smoking and Health Reporter*, Vol. 3, No. 2, p. 3, January 1986.

13. Peter Hersey et al., "Effects of Cigarette Smoking on the Immune System," *Medical Journal of Australia*, Vol. 2, pp. 425-429, October 29, 1983.

14. Kenneth H. Cooper, George O. Gey, Robert A. Bottenberg, "Effects of Cigarette Smoking on Endurance Performance," *Journal of the American Medical Association*, Vol. 203, No. 3, pp. 123-126, January 15, 1968.

15. *The Health Consequences of Smoking: A Report of the Surgeon General*, Chapter 2, p. 11, U.S. Department of Health and Human Services, Washington, DC, 1979.

16. E. C. Hammond, "Life Expectancy of American Men in Relation to Their Smoking Habits," *Journal of the National Cancer Institute*, Vol. 43, pp. 951-962, 1969.

17. *Smoking and Illness*, National Clearinghouse for Smoking and Health, Public Health Service, May 1967.

18. *The Health Consequences of Smoking: Cancer, A Report of the Surgeon General*, U.S. Department of Health and Human Services, Washington, DC, 1982; *Smoking and Illness*, National Clearinghouse for Smoking and Health, Public Health Service, May 1967.

19. *The Health Consequences of Smoking: A Report of the Surgeon General*, Chapter 5, p. 23, U.S. Department of Health and Human Services, Washington, DC, 1979.

20. Ernest L. Wynder, "Tobacco as a Carcinogen," *Your Patient and Cancer*, August 1981, pp. 40-44.

21. Chris Williams, *Lung Cancer: The Facts*, Oxford University Press, New York, 1984, p. 21.

22. Bob Lee, "The Smoldering Cigarette Issue," *Medical World News*, Vol. 24, No. 10, May 23, 1983, pp. 59, 63.

23. "MI Severity in Smokers Proportional to Cumulative Dose of Smoke," *Internal Medicine News*, Vol. 18, No. 4, March 15, 1985.

24. W. B. Kannel, "Prevention of Cardiovascular Disease," *Current Problems in Cardiology*, Vol. 1, pp. 5-68, 1976.

25. Bob Lee, "The Smoldering Cigarette Issue," *Medical World News*, Vol. 24, No. 10, May 23, 1983, p. 59.

26. B. Lawrence Riggs and L. Joseph Melton, "Involutional Osteoporosis," *The New England Journal of Medicine*, Vol. 314, No. 26, pp. 1676-1685, June 26, 1986.

27. Louise A. Brinton et al., "Cigarette Smoking and Invasive Cervical Cancer," *Journal of the American Medical Association*, Vol. 255, No. 23, pp. 3265-3269, June 20, 1986.

28. Jonathan E. Fielding, "Smoking: Health Effects and Control (Part One)," *The New England Journal of Medicine*, Vol. 313, No. 8, August 22, 1985, pp. 491-498.

29. Fielding, pp. 495-496.

30. Ibid.

31. Personal communication (July 10, 1986) from pharmacologist Joe Graedon, author of *The People's Pharmacy* books and the column of the same name.

32. Marianne C. Mierley and Susan P. Baker, "Fatal House Fires in an Urban Population," *Journal of the American Medical Association*, Vol. 249, No. 11, pp. 1466-1468, March 18, 1983.

33. Charles A. Lemaistre, "Nobody Is Safe If a Smoker Is Around," *The New York Times*, January 4, 1987. Michael J. Martin, "Wives of Smokers More Likely to Have Heart Attacks than Wives of Nonsmokers," San Francisco General Hospital (News Release), October 1, 1986. S. Akiba et al., "Passive Smoking and Lung Cancer Among Japanese Women," *World Smoking and Health*, Vol. II, No. 3, Autumn 1986, pp. 4-10.

34. E. Cuyler Hammond, "The Effects of Smoking," *Scientific American*, Vol. 207, No. 1, July 1962.

35. Brian J. Richter and Gio B. Gori, "Demographic and Economic Effects of the Prevention of Early Mortality Associated with Tobacco-Related Diseases," in Gio B. Gori and Fred G. Bock (editors), *A Safe Cigarette?*, Cold Spring Harbor Laboratory, 1980.

36. Jane Brody, "Heart Disease: Big Study Produces New Data," *The New York Times*, January 8, 1985, pp. 17, 20; American Cancer Society, *Dangers of Smoking, Benefits of Quitting, and Relative Risks of Reduced Exposure*, New York, 1980, p. 10; C. P. Howson, *Cigarette Smoking and the Use of Health*

Services, doctoral dissertation, UCLA, 1983, University Microfilms International 84-08815.

37. E. L. Wynder and D. Hoffmann, "Tobacco and Health," *The New England Journal of Medicine*, Vol. 300, pp. 894-903, 1979.

Chapter 4

1. John Urquhart and Klaus Heilmann, *Risk Watch: The Odds of Life*, Facts on File Publications, New York, 1984, pp. 85-90; John Urquhart, personal communication, November 1, 1985.

2. William Poulin, "The Role of the Addictive Process as a Key Step in the Causation of All Tobacco-Related Disease," *The Journal of the American Medical Association*, Vol. 252, No. 20, November 23/30, 1984.

3. Urquhart and Heilmann, pp. xiii.

4. "Health or Smoking?" *British Medical Journal*, Vol. 287, No. 6405, November 26, 1983, pp. 1570-1571.

5. Jack Metcoff et al., "Effect of Food Supplementation (WIC) During Pregnancy on Birth Weight," *The American Journal of Clinical Nutrition*, Vol. 41, pp. 933-947, 1985.

6. Anonymous, "Cigarette Smoking and Spontaneous Abortion," *British Medical Journal*, No. 6108, pp. 259-260, February 4, 1978; Mary Sexton and J. Richard Hebel, "A Clinical Trial of Change in Maternal Smoking and Its Effect on Birth Weight," *The Journal of the American Medical Association*, Vol. 251, No. 7, pp. 911-915, February 17, 1984; Anonymous, "Smoking and Intrauterine Growth," *Lancet*, Vol. 1, pp. 536-537, 1979; M. A. Bureau et al., "Carboxyhemoglobin in Fetal Cord Blood and in Blood of Mothers Who Smoked During Labor," *Pediatrics*, Vol. 69, pp. 371-373; W. A. Divers et al., "Maternal Smoking and Elevation of Catecholamines and Metabolites in the Amniotic Fluid," *The Journal of Obstetrics and Gynecology*, Vol. 141, pp. 625-628, 1981; Figa-Talamanca, "Spontaneous Abortions Among Female Industrial Workers," *Archives of Occupational and Environmental Health*, Vol. 54, No. 2, pp. 163-171, July 1984; J. D. S. Goodman et al., "Effects of Maternal Cigarette Smoking on Fetal Trunk Movements, Fetal Breathing Movements, and Fetal Heart Rate," *British Journal of Obstetrics and Gynecology*, Vol. 91, No. 7, pp. 657-661, July 1984; D. S. Guzick et al., "Predictability of Pregnancy Outcome in

Pre-term Delivery," *Obstetrics and Gynecology*, Vol. 63, No. 5, pp. 645-650, May 1984.

7. Christopher Tietze, "New Estimates of Mortality Associated with Fertility Control," *Family Planning Perspectives*, Vol. 9, No. 2, pp. 74-76, March/April 1977; Samuel Shapiro et al., "Oral Contraceptive Use in Relation to Myocardial Infarction," *Lancet*, Vol. 1, No. 8119, pp. 743-746, April 7, 1979.

8. Paul N. Hopkins, et al., "Magnified Risks from Cigarette Smoking for Coronary Prone Families in Utah," *The Western Journal of Medicine*, Vol. 141, No. 2, pp. 196-202, August 1984; Daniel Pometta et al., "Decreased HDL Cholesterol in Prepubertal and Pubertal Children of CHD Patients," *Atherosclerosis*, Vol. 36, No. 1, pp. 101-109, May 1980.

9. L. E. Daly et al., "Long-term Effect on Mortality of Stopping Smoking After Unstable Angina or Myocardial Infarction," *British Medical Journal*, Vol. 287, No. 6388, pp. 324-326, July 30, 1983; G. B. Cintron, "After the Infarct, What?" *Cardiovascular Reviews and Reports*, Vol. 5, No. 7, pp. 665-668, 671-673, 675-677, July 1984; Stephen Sontag, et al., "Cimetidine, Cigarette Smoking, and Recurrence of Duodenal Ulcer," *The New England Journal of Medicine*, Vol. 311, No. 11, pp. 689-693, September 13, 1984; John M. Elliott, "Cigarettes and Accelerated Hypertension," *The New Zealand Journal of Medicine*, Vol. 91, No. 662, pp. 447-449, June 25, 1980; J. Thomas, "Precursors of Hypertension: A Review," *Journal of the National Medical Association*, Vol. 75, No. 4, pp. 359-369, April 1983; K. W. Beach, et al., "Diabetes and Arteriosclerosis," *Arteriosclerosis*, Vol. 2, p. 275, July/August 1982; F. Lithner, "Is Tobacco of Importance for the Development and Progression of Diabetic Vascular Complications?" *Acta Medica Scandinavica*, Supplement 687, pp. 33-36, 1983; L. Suarez and E. Barrett-Connor, "Interaction Between Cigarette Smoking and Diabetes Mellitus in the Prediction of Death Attributed to Cardiovascular Disease," *American Journal of Epidemiology*, Vol. 120, No. 5, pp. 670-675, November 1984; Harry W. Daniel, "Osteoporosis of the Slender Smoker," *Archives of Internal Medicine*, Vol. 136, March 1976, pp. 298-304; Jytte Jensen et al., "Cigarette Smoking, Serum Estrogens, and Bone Loss During Hormone-Replacement Therapy Early After Menopause," *The New England Journal of Medicine*, Vol. 313, No. 16, pp. 973-975, October 17, 1985; B. Lawrence

Riggs and L. Joseph Melton, "Involutional Osteoporosis," *The New England Journal of Medicine*, Vol. 314, No. 26, pp. 1676-1685, June 26, 1986; H. W. Daniell, "Postmenopausal Tooth Loss: Contributions to Edentulism by Osteoporosis and Cigarette Smoking," *Archives of Internal Medicine*, Vol. 143, No. 9, pp. 1678-1682, September 1983; R. S. Carel et al., "Association Between Ocular Pressure and Certain Health Parameters," *Ophthalmology*, Vol. 91, No. 4, pp. 311-314, April 1984.

10. E. Pukkala et al., "Occupation and Smoking as Risk Determinants of Lung Cancer," *International Journal of Epidemiology*, Vol. 12, No. 3, pp. 290-296, September 1983; B. E. Suta, "Smoking Patterns of Motor Vehicle Industry Workers and Their Impact on Lung Cancer Mortality Rates," *Journal of Occupational Medicine*, Vol. 25, No. 9, pp. 661-667, September 1983; R. G. Ames, "Gastric Cancer and Coal Mine Dust Exposure," *Cancer*, Vol. 52, No. 7, pp. 1346-1350, October 1, 1983; G. A. DoPico et al., "Acute Effects of Grain Dust Exposure During a Work Shift," *American Review of Respiratory Disease*, Vol. 128, No. 3, pp. 399-404, September 1983; J. F. Fraumeni, "The Face of Cancer in the United States," *Hospital Practice*, Vol. 18, No. 12, pp. 81-96, December 1983; G. J. Beck et al., "Cotton Dust and Smoking Effects on Lung Function in Cotton Textile Workers," *American Journal of Epidemiology*, Vol. 119, No. 1, pp. 33-43, January 1984; D. J. Tollerud, et al., "The Health Effects of Automobile Exhaust. VI. Relationship of Respiratory Symptoms and Pulmonary Function in Tunnel and Turnpike Workers," *Archives of Environmental Health*, Vol. 38, No. 6, pp. 334-340, November-December 1983; G. Theriault et al., "Bladder Cancer in the Aluminum Industry," *Lancet*, Vol. 1, No. 8383, pp. 947-950, April 28, 1984; A. Churg and J. L. Wright, "Small Airway Disease and Mineral Dust Exposure," *Pathology Annual*, Vol. 18 (Part 2), pp. 233-251, 1983; Sakari Tola, "Occupational Exposures and Lung Cancer—Epidemiological Approaches," *European Journal of Respiratory Diseases*, Vol. 63, Supplement 123, pp. 128-138, 1982; *Cancer Facts and Figures*, New York, American Cancer Society, February 1984; S. D. Stellman and L. Garfinkel, "Cancer Mortality among Woodworkers," *American Journal of Industrial Medicine*, Vol. 5, No. 5, pp. 343-357, 1984; P. Haglind and R. Rylander, "Exposure to Cotton Dust in an Experimental Cardroom," *British Journal of Industrial Med-*

icine, Vol. 41, No. 3, pp. 340-345, August 1984; M. H. Lloyd et al., "Epidemiological Study of the Lung Function of Workers at a Factory Manufacturing Polyvinylchloride," *British Journal of Industrial Medicine*, Vol. 41, No. 3, pp. 328-333, August 1984; C. Edling and O. Axelson, "Risk Factors of Coronary Heart Disease Among Personnel in a Bus Company," *International Archives of Occupational and Environmental Health*, Vol. 54, No. 2, pp. 181-183, July 1984; C. Laurent et al., "Sister Chromatid Exchange Frequency in Workers Exposed to High Levels of Ethylene Oxide in a Hospital Sterilization Service," *International Archives of Occupational and Environmental Health*, Vol. 54, No. 1, pp. 33-43, April 1984; Maki-Paakkenen et al., "Sister Chromatid Exchanges and Chromosome Aberrations in Rubber Workers," *Teratogenesis, Carcinogenesis, and Mutagenesis*, Vol. 4, No. 2, pp. 189-200, 1984; Council on Scientific Affairs, "A Physician's Guide to Asbestos-related Diseases," *Journal of the American Medical Association*, Vol. 252, No. 18, pp. 2593-2597, November 9, 1984.

11. "The Price of a Paunch," *Medical World News*, February 11, 1985, p. 74; J. Thomas, "Precursors of Hypertension: A Review," *Journal of the National Medical Association*, Vol. 75, No. 4, pp. 359-369, April 1983.

12. Robert J. Garrison et al., "Cigarette Smoking as a Confounder of the Relationship Between Relative Weight and Long-term Mortality," *The Journal of the American Medical Association*, Vol. 249, No. 16, pp. 2199-2203, April 22/29, 1983.

13. H. K. Seitz, "Alkohol und Karzinogenese [Alcohol and Carcinogenesis]", *Leber Magen Darm*, Vol. 12, No. 3, pp. 95-107, 1982; Barry M. Maletzky et al., "Smoking and Alcoholism," *The American Journal of Psychiatry*, Vol. 131, pp. 445-447, 1974; R. Nil, et al., "Effects of Single Doses of Alcohol and Caffeine on Cigarette Smoke Puffing Behavior," *Pharmacology, Biochemistry, and Behavior*, Vol. 20, No. 4, pp. 583-590, April 1984; J. K. Bobo and L. D. Gilchrist, "Urging the Alcoholic Client to Quit Smoking," *Addictive Behaviors*, Vol. 8, No. 3, pp. 297-305, 1983.

14. R. Nil et al., "The Smoker, His Smoking Behavior, and His Motivation for Smoking," *Psychologie*, Vol. 41, No. 2, pp. 217-229, 1982.

15. Jane Brody, "Those Most Likely to Light Up," *The New York Times*, January 15, 1984, p. 6E.

16. J. B. Jobe et al., "Risk Taking as Motivation for Volunteering for a Hazardous Experiment," *Journal of Personality*, Vol. 51, No. 1, pp. 95-107, March 1983.

17. P. Grout et al., "Cigarette Smoking, Road Traffic Accidents, and Seat Belt Usage," *Public Health*, Vol. 97, No. 2, pp. 95-101, March 1983.

18. Meyer Friedman and Diane Ulmer, *Treating Type A Behavior—and Your Heart*, Alfred A. Knopf, New York, 1984.

19. J. R. Kabam et al., Vanderbilt University Hospital, a Presentation at the annual meeting of the American Society of Anesthesiologists, reported in *American Family Physician*, November 1982; P. Layde, "Risk Factors for Complications of Interval Tubal Sterilization by Laparotomy," *Obstetrics and Gynecology*, Vol. 62, No. 2, pp. 180-184, August 1984.

20. J. Thomas, "Precursors of Hypertension: A Review," *Journal of the National Medical Association*, Vol. 75, No. 4, pp. 359-369, April 1983.

21. David Sobel and Tom Ferguson, *The People's Book of Medical Tests*, Summit Books, New York, 1985, p. 149.

22. M. C. Zaslow, "Human Neutrophil Elastase Does Not Bind to Alpha-One Protease Inhibitor That Has Been Exposed to Activated Human Neutrophils," *American Review of Respiratory Disease*, Vol. 128, No. 3, pp. 434-439, September 1983.

23. Alan R. Dyer et al., "Heart Rate as a Prognostic Factor for Coronary Heart Disease and Mortality," *American Journal of Epidemiology*, Vol. 112, No. 6, 1980, pp. 736-749.

24. Blanco Licina Cedres et al., "Independent Contribution of Electrocardiographic (EKG) Abnormalities to Risk of Death from Coronary Heart Disease and All Causes," *Circulation*, Vol. 65, No. 1, pp. 146-153, January 1982.

25. Paul D. Sorlie, "Hematocrit and Risk of Coronary Heart Disease," *American Heart Journal*, Vol. 101, No. 4, April 1981, pp. 456-461.

26. Lynn T. Koslowski et al., "Tobacco Dependence, Restraint, and Time to the First Cigarette of the Day," *Addictive Behaviors*, Vol. 6, pp. 307-312, 1981; "Smoker's Quiz Shows Degree of Addiction," *The Fitness Bulletin*, Vol. 7, No. 9, September 1984, p. 2.

Chapter 5

1. Arden G. Christen and Kenneth H. Cooper, "Strategic Withdrawal from Cigarette Smoking," *CA: A Cancer Journal for Clinicians*, Vol. 29, No. 2, pp. 96-107, March/April 1979. Dr. Pomerleau's comments are quoted from Robert Kanigel and Tom Yulsman, "By Smoke Possessed," *American Health*, June 1986, pp. 43-47.

2. The Gallup Organization, "Public Attitudes and Behavior Related to Exercise," poll conducted for *American Health* magazine, November, 1984.

3. John D. Kaufman, "Stopping Smoking," *The New England Journal of Medicine*, Vol. 301, No. 7, p. 389, August 16, 1979.

4. J. S. Hill, *Effect of a Program of Aerobic Exercise on the Smoking Behavior of a Group of Adult Volunteers*, doctoral dissertation, Ohio State University, 1982, University Microfilms International No. 83-05340.

5. S. N. Blair, N. N. Goodyear, K. L. Wynne, et al., "Comparison of Dietary and Smoking Habit Changes in Physical Fitness Improvers and Nonimprovers," *Preventive Medicine*, Vol. 13, No. 4, pp. 411-420, July 1984.

6. Peter Wood, "Living the Good Life is a Business That Can Kill," *San Francisco Examiner*, October 6, 1985, pp. B-1 & B-2.

7. Christen and Cooper, op. cit.

8. F. Heinzelmann and R. W. Bagley, "Response to Physical Activity Programs and Their Effects on Health Behavior," *Public Health Reports*, Vol. 85, pp. 905-911, 1970.

9. Ralph S. Paffenbarger, Robert T. Hyde, Alvin L. Wing, Charles H. Steinmetz, "A Natural History of Athleticism and Cardiovascular Health," *Journal of the American Medical Association*, Vol. 252, No. 4, pp. 491-495, July 27, 1984; Paffenbarger et al., "Physical Activity, All-Cause Mortality, and Longevity of College Alumni," *The New England Journal of Medicine*, Vol. 314, No. 10, pp. 605-613, March 6, 1986; Jane Brody, "Study Indicates Moderate Exercise Can Add Years to a Person's Life," *The New York Times*, March 6, 1986, pp. 1, 15.

10. The table comparing risks of death for smokers and nonsmokers by exercise level is adapted from E. Cuyler Hammond, "Smoking in Relation to Mortality and Morbidity,"

Journal of the National Cancer Institute, Vol. 32, pp. 1161-1188, May 1964.

11. Kenneth H. Cooper, *Running Without Fear: How to Reduce the Risk of Heart Attack and Sudden Death During Aerobic Exercise*, M. Evans, New York, 1985, p. 185.

12. George Sheehan, personal communication, July 1983.

13. Linn Goldberg, Diane L. Elliot, Ronald W. Schultz, and Frank E. Kloster, "Changes in Lipid and Lipoprotein Levels After Weight Training, *Journal of the American Medical Association*, Vol. 252, No. 4, July 27, 1984, pp. 504-506.

14. Committee on Diet, Nutrition, and Cancer of the National Research Council of the National Academy of Sciences, *Diet, Nutrition, and Cancer*, National Academy Press, Washington, DC, 1982, pp. 14-16.

15. Takeshi Hirayama, "Changing Patterns of Cancer in Japan with Special Reference to the Decrease in Stomach Cancer Mortality," in H. H. Hiatt et al., *Origins of Human Cancer, Book A: Incidence of Cancer in Humans*, Cold Spring Harbor Laboratory, Cold Spring Harbor, NY, 1977, pp. 55-75.

16. This jingle has been adapted from a similar jingle by Michael Jacobson, director of The Center for Science in the Public Interest in Washington, DC; Tom Ferguson, "A Field Guide to Eating: A Conversation with Michael Jacobson," in *Medical Self-Care: Access to Health Tools*, Summit Books, 1980, pp. 137-142.

17. Carole Bullock, "Fruits and Veges Cut Oral, Pharyngeal Ca Risk," *Medical Tribune*, May 2, 1984; Wang Long-de, and E. Cuyler Hammond, "Lung Cancer, Fruit, Green Salad, and Vitamin Pills," *Chinese Medical Journal*, Vol. 98, No. 3, pp. 206-211, 1985.

18. Bonnie F. Lieberman and Michael F. Jacobson, "Anti-Cancer Eating Guide," *Healthline*, Vol. 5, No. 2, March 1986, pp. 8-9.

19. U. Saffiotti et al., "Experimental Cancer of the Lung," *Cancer*, Vol. 20, No. 5, pp. 857-864, 1967; J. Gouveia et al., "Degree in Bronchial Metaplasia in Heavy Smokers and Its Regression After Treatment with a Retinoid," *Lancet*, March 27, 1982, pp. 710-712; Gunnar Kvale et al., "Dietary Habits and Lung Cancer Risk," *International Journal of Cancer*, Vol. 31, pp. 397-405, 1983; E. Bjelke, "Dietary Vitamin A and Human Lung Cancer," *International Journal of Cancer*, Vol. 15, pp. 561-565, 1975; Michael B. Sporn, "Chemoprevention of Cancer," *Nature*, Vol. 272, pp. 402-403, 1978;

Carlo Lavecchia et al., "Dietary Vitamin A and the Risk of Cervical Cancer," *International Journal of Cancer*, Vol. 34, pp. 319-322, 1984; Michael B. Sporn, "Retinoids and Carcinogenesis," *Nutrition Reviews*, Vol. 35, No. 4, pp. 65-69, 1977.

20. Sheldon Saul Hendler, *The Complete Guide to Anti-Aging Nutrients*, Simon & Schuster, New York, 1985, p. 85.

21. Joe Graedon, personal communication, March 1986.

22. R. J. Waski, "Vitamin C and Smoking," presented at the Fifth World Congress on Smoking and Health, Winnipeg, Canada, July 10-15, 1983, reported in *ASH Review*, November 1983, p. 6; Omer Pelletier, "Vitamin C Status of Cigarette Smokers and Nonsmokers," *American Journal of Clinical Nutrition*, Vol. 23, No. 5, May 1970, pp. 520-524; "One Cigarette Destroys the Amount of Vitamin C That is Found in One Orange," *Smoking and Health Review*, Action for Smoking and Health, November 1982, p. 12; L. R. Shapiro et al., "Patterns of Vitamin C Intake from Food and Supplements," *American Journal of Public Health*, Vol. 73, No. 7, pp. 773-778, July 1983.

23. Bruce Ames, "Dietary Carcinogens and Anticarcinogens," *Science*, Vol. 221, pp. 1256-1264, September 23, 1983; Committee on Diet, Nutrition, and Cancer, *Diet, Nutrition, and Cancer*, The National Research Council of the National Academy of Sciences, National Academy Press, Washington, DC, 1982, pp. 163-169.

24. Ames, op. cit.; Hendler, *The Complete Guide to Anti-Aging Nutrients*, pp. 176-185; Bonnie Liebman, "Selenium: Must We Rely on Supplements to Get Enough?" *Nutrition Action*, Vol. 10, No. 10, December 1983, pp. 5-10; "Daily Selenium Supplement Caused Toxic Effects," *Family Practice News*, Vol. 15, No. 14, July 15-31, 1985.

25. W. S. Foulds et al., "Vitamin B-12 Absorption in Tobacco Amblyopia," *British Journal of Ophthalmology*, Vol. 53, pp. 393-397, 1969; J. C. Linnell et al., "Effects of Smoking on Metabolism and Excretion of Vitamin B-12," *British Medical Journal*, Vol. 2, pp. 215-216, April 1968; Hendler, *The Complete Guide to Anti-Aging Nutrients*, pp. 102-104.

26. Committee on Diet, Nutrition, and Cancer of the National Research Council of the National Academy of Sciences, *Diet, Nutrition, and Cancer*, National Academy Press, Washington, DC, 1982, p. 362.

27. Personal communication, Sheldon Saul Hendler, M.D., Uni-

versity of California School of Medicine, San Diego, June 9, 1986.

28. *Diet, Nutrition, and Cancer*, pp. 130-137; Bonnie F. Liebman and Michael F. Jacobson, "Anti-Cancer Eating Guide," *Healthline*, Vol. 5, No. 2, March 1986, pp. 8-9.

29. Hendler, op. cit.

30. *Diet, Nutrition, and Cancer*, pp. 92-93.

31. "60% to 80% of All Industrial Accidents Are Related to Stress," *Internal Medicine News*, Vol. 18, No. 18, September 15-30, 1985.

32. Alan Lakein, *How to Get Control of Your Time and Your Life*, Signet, New York, 1973.

33. For a free catalog of inexpensive time-planning notebooks, write Daytimers, Inc., Allentown, PA 18001, (215) 395-5884. For a more expensive top-of-the-line planning notebook, send for information on the Time/Design system: Time/Design, 2101 Wilshire Blvd., Santa Monica, CA 90403, (800) 637-9942.

34. The advice on dealing effectively with stress was excerpted from several long discussions between Dr. Pelletier and the author. An earlier version of this material appeared in Tom Ferguson, "Do-It-Yourself Stress Relief: A Conversation with Kenneth R. Pelletier, Ph.D.," *Medical Self-Care*, No. 36, September 1986.

35. Christen and Cooper, p. 106.

36. J. L. Schwartz and G. Rider, "Smoking Cessation Methods in the United States and Canada, 1969-1974," in *Smoking and Health: Proceedings of the Third World Conference*, 1975, Washington, DC, U.S. Department of Health, Education, and Welfare, 1975.

37. Ovide Pomerleau and Cynthia S. Pomerleau, *Break the Smoking Habit: A Behavioral Program for Giving Up Cigarettes*, Behavioral Medicine Press, West Hartford, CT, 1977.

38. Wayne Glad and Vincent J. Adesso, "The Relative Importance of Socially Induced Tension and Behavioral Cognition for Smoking Behavior," *Journal of Abnormal Psychology*, Vol. 85, pp. 119-121, 1976.

39. Pomerleau and Pomerleau, op. cit., pp. 13-14.

40. S. Leonard Syme and Rina Alcalay, "Control of Cigarette Smoking from a Social Perspective," *Annual Review of Public Health*, Vol. 3, pp. 179-199, 1982.

41. Jack Stiggins, "Freedom Line: Increasing Utilization of a

Telephone Support Service for Ex-Smokers," *Addictive Behaviors*, Vol. 9, pp. 227-230, 1984.

Chapter 6

1. Lee W. Frederiksen, "Controlled Smoking," in N. A. Krasnegor (editor), *Behavioral Analysis and Treatment of Substance Abuse*, NIDA Research Monograph No. 25, June 1979, DHEW Publication No. (ADM) 79-839.

2. Personal communication from Russell E. Glasgow, June 13, 1986.

3. Russell E. Glasgow, Robert C. Klesges, Phillip R. Godding, and Randy Gegelman, "Controlled Smoking, With and Without Carbon Monoxide Feedback, as an Alternative for Chronic Smokers," *Behavior Therapy*, Vol. 14, pp. 386-397, 1983; Russell E. Glasgow, Robert C. Klesges, Lisa M. Klesges, Michael W. Vasey, and Daniel F. Gunnarson, "Long-term Effects of a Controlled Smoking Program: A $2\frac{1}{2}$ Year Follow-Up," *Behavior Therapy*, Vol. 16, pp. 303-307, 1985; L. W. Frederiksen, G. L. Peterson, and W. D. Murphy, "Controlled Smoking, Development and Maintenance," *Addictive Behaviors*, Vol. 1, pp. 193-196, 1976.

4. Personal communication from Russell E. Glasgow, June 13, 1986.

5. Glasgow, Klesges, Godding, and Gegelman, op. cit.

6. Edward Lichtenstein and David O. Antonuccio, "Dimensions of Smoking Behavior," *Addictive Behaviors*, Vol. 6, pp. 365-367, 1981; Lee W. Frederiksen, Peter M. Miller, and Gerald L. Peterson, "Topographical Components of Smoking Behavior," *Addictive Behaviors*, Vol. 2, pp. 55-61, 1977.

7. D. O. Ho-Yen et al., "Why Smoke Fewer Cigarettes?" *British Medical Journal*, Vol. 284, pp. 1905-1907, June 26, 1982; M. A. H. Russell et al., *British Journal of Addiction*, Vol. 77, p. 145, July 1982.

8. E. Cuyler Hammond, "The Effects of Smoking," *Scientific American*, Vol. 207, No. 1, P. 47, July 1962.

9. Tim Higenbottam et al., "Cigarette Smoke Inhalation and the Acute Airway Response," *Thorax*, Vol. 35, No. 4. pp. 246-254, 1980.

10. Barbara Stephens Brockway et al., "Non-Aversive Procedures and Their Effect on Cigarette Smoking," *Addictive Behaviors*, Vol. 2, pp. 121-128, 1977.

11. Arden G. Christen and Kenneth H. Cooper, "Strategic With-

drawal from Cigarette Smoking,'' *CA: A Cancer Journal for Clinicians*, Vol. 29, No. 2, March/April 1979, pp. 96-107.

12. Personal communication from Alice Kahn, June 1983.

13. Ovide F. Pomerleau and Cynthia S. Pomerleau, *Break the Smoking Habit: A Behavioral Program for Giving Up Cigarettes*, Behavioral Medicine Press, West Hartford, CT, 1977.

14. Personal communication from Richard L. Miller, Ph.D., September 1981.

Chapter 7

1. Office of Smoking and Health, personal communication, May 1986.

2. W. S. Rikert, '' 'Less Hazardous' Cigarettes: Fact or Fiction?'' *New York State Journal of Medicine*, Vol. 83, No. 13, pp. 1269-1272, December 1983; M. Llanos, "Improvements in Reducing Risks to Smokers," *Tabak Journal International*, Vol. 4, No. 266, pp. 268-269, August 1983.

3. Rickert, op. cit.; Llanos, op. cit.; J. Rimington, "Cigarette Filters and Lung Cancer," *Environmental Research*, Vol. 24, pp. 162-166, 1981, reprinted in *World Smoking and Health*, Spring 1982, pp. 38-42; J. H. Lutschg, "Why Uncle Sam Is Still Smoking," *New York State Journal of Medicine*, Vol. 83, No. 13, pp. 1278-1279, 1983; N. Benowitz et al., "Smokers of Low-Yield Cigarettes Do Not Consume Less Nicotine," *New England Journal of Medicine*, Vol. 309, No. 3, pp. 139-142, July 21, 1983.

4. Ernest L. Wynder, "Tobacco as a Carcinogen," *Your Patient & Cancer*, August 1981, pp. 40-44.

5 William P. Castelli et al., "The Filter Cigarette and Coronary Heart Disease: The Framingham Study," *Lancet*, Vol. 2, No. 8238, pp. 109-113, July 18, 1981; David W. Kaufman, "Constituents of Cigarette Smoke and Cardiovascular Disease," *New York State Journal of Medicine*, December 1983, pp. 1267-1268; David W. Kaufman et al., "Nicotine and Carbon Monoxide Content of Cigarette Smoke and the Risk of Myocardial Infarction in Young Men," *The New England Journal of Medicine*, Vol. 308, No. 8, pp. 409-413, February 24, 1983; *The Health Consequences of Smoking: The Changing Cigarette*. A Report of the Surgeon General, U.S. Department of Health and Human Services, 1981, p. 120; E. C. Hammond, "The Long-term Benefits of Reducing Tar and Nicotine in Cigarettes," in G. B. Gori and F. G. Bock, *A Safe Cigarette?*,

Branbury Report No. 3, Cold Spring Harbor Laboratory, Cold Spring Harbor, NY, 1980; The Surgeon General, "Smoking and Cancer," in *Morbidity and Mortality Weekly Reports*, Vol. 31, pp. 77-80, 1982.

6. C. Lenfant, "Are 'Low-Yield' Cigarettes Really Safer?" *New England Journal of Medicine*, Vol. 309, No. 3, pp. 181-182, July 21, 1983; R. V. Ebert et al., "Amount of Nicotine and Carbon Monoxide Inhaled by Smokers of Low-Tar, Low-Nicotine Cigarettes," *Journal of the American Medical Association*, Vol. 250, No. 20, pp. 2840-2842; W. S. Rickert, " 'Less Hazardous' Cigarettes: Fact or Fiction?" *New York State Journal of Medicine*, Vol. 83, No. 13, pp. 1269-1272, December 1983.

7. E. C. Hammond et al., "Tar and Nicotine Content of Cigarette Smoke in Relation to Death Rates," *Environmental Research*, Vol. 12, pp. 263-274, 1976; Hammond, "The Long-term Benefits of Reducing Tar and Nicotine in Cigarettes," op. cit.

8. D. J. Weeks and S. P. Todd, "Cigarette Tar Cheat," *New Scientist*, Vol. 99, No. 1370, p. 431, August 11, 1983.

9. Rickert, " 'Less Hazardous' Cigarettes: Fact or Fiction?" op. cit.

10. "The Ultra-Low-Tar Gimmick," *Consumer Reports*, January 1983, pp. 26-27, 50.

11. Weeks and Todd, op. cit.; T. Lombardo et al., "When Low-Tar Cigarettes Yield High Tar: Cigarette Filter Ventilation Hole Blocking and Its Detection," *Addictive Behaviors*, Vol. 8, No. 1, pp. 67-69, 1983; D. Hoffmann, J. D. Adams, and N. J. Haley, "Reported Cigarette Smoke Values, A Closer Look," *American Journal of Public Health*, Vol. 73, No. 9, pp. 1050-1053, September 1983.

12. *Consumer Reports*, op. cit.

13. S. R. Sutton et al., "Relationship Between Cigarette Yields, Puffing Patterns, and Smoke Intake: Evidence for Tar Compensation," *British Medical Journal*, Vol. 285, August 28-September 4, 1982, pp. 600-603; M. A. H. Russell et al., "Long-term Switching to Low-Tar, Low-Nicotine Cigarettes," *British Journal of Addiction*, Vol. 77, pp. 145-158, 1982; "Milder Cigarettes Don't Reduce the Hazards," *Medical World News*, October 11, 1982.

14. E. C. Hammond and D. Horn, "Smoking and Death Rates—Report on Forty-Four Months of Follow-Up of 187,783 Men," *Journal of the American Medical Association*, Vol. 166, pp.

1294-1308, March 15, 1958, reprinted in *Journal of the American Medical Association*, Vol. 251, No. 21, pp. 2840-2853, June 1, 1984.

15. R. Doll, "Smoking and Death Rates," *Journal of the American Medical Association*, Vol. 251, No. 21, pp. 2854-2857, June 1, 1984; R. V. Ebert and M. E. McNabb, "Cessation of Smoking in Prevention and Treatment of Cardiac and Pulmonary Disease," *Archives of Internal Medicine*, Vol. 144, No. 8, pp. 1558ff, August 1984; M. A. H. Russell, "Realistic Goals for Smoking and Health," *Lancet*, February 16, 1974, pp. 254-257; K. McCusker et al., "Physical Properties of Smoke from Cigarettes Compared to Pipes," *Chest*, Vol. 78, No. 2, p. 530, September 1980.

16. J. H. Lubin, B. S. Richter, and W. J. Blot, "Lung Cancer Risk with Cigar and Pipe Use," *Journal of the National Cancer Institute*, Vol. 73, No. 2, pp. 377-381, August 1984.

17. "Warning: Inhaled Cigar Smoke May Be Particularly Hazardous," *Journal of the American Medical Association*, Vol. 232, No. 13, pp. 1319-1320, June 30, 1975.

18. S. W. Byrne, *Filtering Means*, U.S. Patent Number 4,481,959, November 13, 1984.

19. T. Yamaguchi, *Cigarette Filter*, U.S. Patent Number 31,700, October 9, 1984.

20. John D. Bogden et al., "Relatively High Selenium Concentrations in Cigarette Tobaccos from Low Lung Cancer Incidence Countries," *Federation Proceedings*, Vol. 39, No. 3, Part 1, March 1, 1980, p. 556; Bogden et al., "Selenium, Tar, and Nicotine Concentrations of Cigarette Tobaccos from Low Lung Cancer Incidence Countries," *American Review of Respiratory Disease*, Vol. 121, No. 4, Part 2, April 1980, p. 224.

21. N. H. Harley and B. S. Cohen, "Polonium 210: A Questionable Risk Factor in Smoking-Related Carcinogenesis," in G. B. Gori and F. G. Bock, *A Safe Cigarette?*, Branbury Report No. 3, Cold Spring Harbor Laboratory, Cold Spring Harbor, NY, 1980.

Chapter 8

1. The following publications were important overall sources for this chapter: Russell E. Glasgow, "Smoking," in *Self-Management of Chronic Disease*, K. Holoroyd and T. Cheer (editors), Academic Press, New York, 1985; Arden G. Chris-

ten and Kenneth H. Cooper, ''Strategic Withdrawal from Cigarette Smoking,'' *CA: A Cancer Journal for Clinicians*, Vol. 29, No. 2, pp. 96-107, March/April 1979; Brian G. Danaher and Edward Lichtenstein, *Become an Ex-Smoker*, Prentice-Hall, Englewood Cliffs, NJ, 1978.

2. John W. Farquhar, ''How to Stop Smoking,'' *Medical Self-Care*, No. 7, Winter 1979/1980, pp. 38-49; Jerome L. Schwartz, *Review and Evaluation of Smoking Cessation Methods: The United States and Canada, 1978-1984*, National Cancer Institute, Bethesda, Maryland, 1986; Personal communication from Jerome L. Schwartz, April 1986.

3. E. E. Levitt, ''Smoking Withdrawal: An Evaluation of Its Role in the Total Effort to Eliminate Smoking,'' presented at the Fifth World Conference on Smoking and Health, abstracted in *Smoking and Health Reporter*, November 1983, p. 7; Jerome L. Schwartz, *Review and Evaluation of Smoking Cessation Methods: The United States and Canada, 1978-1984*, National Cancer Institute, Bethesda, Maryland, 1986; personal communication from Jerome L. Schwartz, March 1986.

4. Personal communication from Frank Reissman, January 1986.

5. Jackie C. Wood, ''Stopping Smoking: What the Experts Say,'' *Healthline*, December 1983, p. 5.

6. Jerome L. Schwartz, *Review and Evaluation of Smoking Cessation Methods: The United States and Canada, 1978-1984*, National Cancer Institute, Bethesda, Maryland, 1986.

7. Stanley Schachter, ''Don't Sell Habit-Breakers Short,'' *Psychology Today*, August 1982, pp. 27-33; Stanley Schachter, ''Self-Treatment of Smoking and Obesity,'' *Canadian Journal of Public Health*, Vol. 72, No. 6, pp. 401-406, November/December 1981. Comparing Dr. Schachter's figures with those of smoking cessation clinics can be somewhat misleading—his figures represent a cumulative percentage, while the clinic figures represent a single trial. The conclusion to be drawn here is not that do-it-yourself methods are superior to clinic methods, but that smokers who are determined to quit stand a good chance of being successful in the long run.

8. The ten stages of quitting presented here were developed by the author, based in part on the five stages of quitting (precontemplation, contemplation, action, maintenance, and relapse) as described by James O. Prochaska and Carlo C. DiClemente in ''Stages and Processes of Self-Change of

Smoking,'' *Journal of Consulting and Clinical Psychology*, Vol. 51, No. 3, pp. 390-395, 1983.

9. Personal communication from Saul Shiffman, Assistant Professor of Psychology, University of Pittsburgh, June 13, 1986.

10. M. G. Perry and C. S. Richards, ''An Investigation of Naturally Occurring Episodes of Self-Controlled Behaviors, *The Journal of Consulting Psychology*, Vol. 24, pp. 178-183, 1977; M. G. Perry et al., ''Behavioral Self-Control and Smoking Reduction: A Study of Self-Initiated Attempts to Reduce Smoking,'' *Behavior Therapy*, Vol. 8, pp. 360-365, 1977.

11. Jackie C. Wood, ''Stopping Smoking: What the Experts Say,'' *Healthline*, Vol. 2, No. 12, December 1983, p. 5.

12. Robert C. Benfari, quoted in ''Three Factors Seem to Predict Inability to Give Up Smoking,'' *Internal Medicine News*, Vol. 15, No. 24, December 15-31, 1982.

13. Judith K. Ockene et al., ''Relationship of Psychological Factors to Smoking Behavior Change in an Intervention Program,'' *Preventive Medicine*, Vol. 11, No. 1, pp. 13-28, 1982.

14. John S. Tamerin, ''The Psychodynamics of Quitting Smoking in a Group,'' *American Journal of Psychiatry*, Vol. 129, No. 5, pp. 101, 104, November 1972; Victor Strecher, ''Want to Quit Smoking? Believe in Yourself, Temple Prof Says,'' news release, Temple University, Philadelphia, PA, October 13, 1983; S. T. Tiffany, *Treatments for Cigarette Smoking*, doctoral dissertation, University of Wisconsin, Madison, August 1984, University Microfilms International 84-1972.

15. Z. S. Ashenberg, *Smoking Recidivism: The Role of Stress and Coping*, doctoral dissertation, Department of Psychology, Washington University, St. Louis, August 1983, University Microfilms International 84-02189.

16. The quote from Dr. Jaffee appeared in Robert Kanigel and Tom Yulsman, ''By Smoke Possessed,'' *American Health*, June 1986, pp. 43-47.

17. Personal communication from Saul Shiffman, June 13, 1986.

18. Ibid.

19. Adapted from John W. Farquhar, ''How to Stop Smoking,'' in *Medical Self-Care*, No. 7, Winter 1979/80, pp. 39-49.

20. Saul Shiffman, ''A Cluster-Analytic Classification of Smoking Relapse Situations,'' *Addictive Behaviors*, Vol. 11, 1986 (in press).

21. Glen D. Morgan and E. B. Fisher, ''Influences of Friends, Spouse, and Family in Maintenance of Smoking Cessation,''

presented at the annual meeting of the Society of Behavioral Medicine, May 23-26, 1984.

22. Robin Mermelstein, Edward Lichtenstein, and Karen McIntyre, "Partner Support and Relapse in Smoking-Cessation Programs," *Journal of Consulting and Clinical Psychology*, Vol. 51, No. 3, pp. 465-466, 1983; H. Catherina Coppotelli and C. Tracy Orleans, "Spouse Support for Smoking Cessation Maintenance by Women," presented at the annual meeting of the Society of Behavioral Medicine, May 23-26, 1984.

23. Irving L. Janis, "The Role of Social Support in Adherence to Stressful Decisions," *American Psychologist*, February 1983, pp. 143-160. Edward Lichtenstein comments: "The results of the Janis study suggest that after ten years, the smoking rate among members of the high-contact buddy group was *less than one-twentieth* that of the control group. No other researchers to date have been able to replicate these striking results" (personal communication from Edward Lichtenstein, Professor of Psychology, University of Oregon, Eugene).

24. Olvide Pomerleau, David Adkins, and Michael Pertschuk, "Predictors of Outcome and Recidivism in Smoking Cessation Treatment," *Addictive Behaviors*, Vol. 3, pp. 65-70, 1978.

25. R. C. Gunn, "Does Living With Smokers Make Quitting Cigarettes More Difficult?" *Addictive Behaviors*, Vol. 8, No. 4, pp. 429-432, 1983.

26. Dr. Sach's conclusions are cited in "No Sure Thing Among Stop-Smoking Plans," *Medical World News*, December 23, 1985, p. 51, and "Short, Intense Counseling Can Get Smokers to Quit," *Family Practice News*, Vol. 14, No. 19, October 1-14, 1984, p. 10.

27. Arden G. Christen and Kenneth H. Cooper, "Strategic Withdrawal from Cigarette Smoking," *CA: A Cancer Journal for Clinicians*, Vol. 29, No. 2, March/April 1979, p. 105.

28. Irving L. Janis and Leon Mann, "Effectiveness of Emotional Role-playing in Modifying Smoking Habits and Attitudes," *Journal of Experimental Research in Personality*, Vol. 1, pp. 84-90, 1965.

29. David L. Geisinger, *Kicking It: The New Way to Stop Smoking Permanently*, New American Library, New York, 1978, pp. 82-84.

30. Saul M. Shiffman, "The Tobacco Withdrawal Syndrome," in

Norman A. Krasnegor (editor), *Cigarette Smoking as a Dependence Process*, NIDA Research Monograph #23, January 1979, National Institute on Drug Abuse, pp. 158-184.

31. Nina G. Schneider and Murray E. Jarvik, "Time Course of Smoking Withdrawal Symptoms as a Function of Nicotine Replacement," *Psychopharmacology*, Vol. 82, pp. 143-144, 1984.

32. G. Alan Marlatt, "Cognitive Factors in the Relapse Process," in G. Alan Marlatt and Judith R. Gordon (editors), *Relapse Prevention: Maintenance Strategies in the Treatment of Addictive Behaviors*, The Guilford Press, New York, 1985.

33. If you do find that you've made a major slip, Dr. John Farquhar of Stanford University suggests the following:

1. Temporarily seek to lower your health risk by other means (exercise program, eating or stress reduction, cutting down or stopping alcohol and/or caffeine consumption, etc.) before attempting to quit smoking again.

2. Smoke the smallest number of cigarettes you can.

3. Review the brand-switching strategies for dose reduction. Look ahead to a future opportunity to quit altogether.

Above all, don't lose heart. Studies suggest that having tried to quit in the past increases your chances of succeeding the next time. See John W. Farquhar, "How to Stop Smoking," in *Medical Self-Care*, No. 7, Winter 1979-80, pp. 39-49.

34. Saul Shiffman et al., "Preventing Relapse in Ex-Smokers: A Self-Management Approach," in Marlatt and Gordon, op cit.

35. M. A. H. Russell, "Comments," in Gio B. Gori and Fred G. Bock (editors), *A Safe Cigarette?* Cold Spring Harbor Laboratory, 1980, p. 296; R. M. Gilbert and M. A. Pope, "Early Effects of Quitting Smoking," *Psychopharmacology*, Vol. 78, No. 2, pp. 121-127, October 1982.

36. Drs. Auerbach, Castelli, and Cahan are quoted in "The Smoldering Cigarette Issue: How Can Your Patients Quit?" *Medical World News*, Vol. 24, No. 10, pp. 43-63, May 23, 1983. See also Betty Kirk, "Smokers: It's Not Too Late to Revitalize Your Immune System," *UTCHS Medical Journal*, August 31, 1984, p. 1.

37. R. I. Levy, "Causes of the Decrease in Cardiovascular Mortality," *American Journal of Cardiology*, Vol. 54, No. 5, pp. 7C-13C, August 27, 1984.

38. J. H. Lubin et al., "Modifying Risk of Developing Lung Cancer by Changing Habits of Cigarette Smoking," *British*

Medical Journal, Vol. 228, No. 6435, pp. 1953-1956, June 30, 1984.

Chapter 9

1. Neal L. Benowitz, "Clinical Pharmacology of Nicotine," in *Annual Review of Medicine*, 1986 (in press); John Grabowski and Sharon M. Hall, "Tobacco Use, Treatment Strategies, and Pharmacological Adjuncts: An Overview," in *Pharmacological Adjuncts in Smoking Cessation*, John Grabowski and Sharon M. Hall (editors), NIDA Research Monograph #53, National Institute on Drug Abuse, 1985, p. 8.
2. Personal communication from M. A. H. Russell, June 12, 1986.
3. M. A. H. Russell and M. J. Jarvis, "Theoretical Background and Clinical Use of Nicotine Chewing Gum," in *Pharmacological Adjuncts in Smoking Cessation*, Grabowski and Hall, p. 126.
4. Ibid., p. 116.
5. B. Brantmark et al., "Nicotine-Containing Chewing Gum as an Anti-Smoking Aid," *Psychopharmacologia* (Berlin), Vol. 31, pp. 191-200, 1973; Ove Ferno, "A Substitute for Tobacco Smoking" (Nicotine Chewing Gum), *Psychopharmacologia* (Berlin), Vol. 31, pp. 201-204, 1973; U.S. Food and Drug Administration New Drug Application #18-612, Nicotine Resin Complex (Nicorette), March 17, 1981, Merrill-Dow Pharmaceuticals, Inc., Cincinnati, Ohio; Nicorette Package Insert, Merrill-Dow, 1984; Norman L. Jacobson et al., "Non-Combustible Cigarette: Alternative Method of Delivery," *Chest*, Vol. 76, No. 3, September 1979, pp. 355-356; J. E. Rose et al., "Transdermal Administration of Nicotine" (Nicotine Skin Patch), *Drug and Alcohol Dependence*, Vol. 13, pp. 209-213, 1984; R. Stepney, "Why Do People Smoke?" (Nicotine Inhaler), *New Society*, Vol. 85, No. 1080, pp. 126-128, July 28, 1983; M. A. H. Russell et al., "Theoretical Background and Clinical Use of Nicotine Chewing Gum" (Nicotine Chewing Gum, Nicotine Lozenges, Nicotine Tablets, Nicotine Suppositories, Nicotine Pessaries, Nicotine Injections, and Nasal Nicotine Solution or "Liquid Snuff"), *Pharmacological Adjuncts in Smoking Cessation*, Grabowski and Hall, pp. 110-130.
6. M. J. Jarvis et al., "Randomized Controlled Trial of Nicotine

Chewing-Gum," *British Medical Journal*, Vol. 285, pp. 537-540, August 21, 1982.

7. M. J. Jarvis et al., "Randomized Controlled Trial of Nicotine Chewing-Gum," *British Medical Journal*, Vol. 285, pp. 537-540, August 21, 1982; John R. Hughes and Dorothy Hatsukami, "Short-Term Effects of Nicotine Gum," in *Pharmacological Adjuncts in Smoking Cessation*, Grabowski and Hall, pp. 70-74; Nina G. Schneider and Murray E. Jarvik, "Nicotine Gum vs. Placebo Gum: Comparisons of Withdrawal Symptoms and Success Rates," in *Pharmacological Adjuncts in Smoking Cessation*, Grabowski and Hall, pp. 83-101.

8. M. A. H. Russell and M. J. Jarvis, "Theoretical Background and Clinical Use of Nicotine Chewing Gum," in *Pharmacological Adjuncts in Smoking Cessation*, Grabowski and Hall, pp. 110-130.

9. Karl-Olov Fagerstrom and Bo Melin, "Nicotine Chewing Gum in Smoking Cessation: Efficiency, Nicotine Dependence, Therapy Duration, and Clinical Recommendations," in *Pharmacological Adjuncts in Smoking Cessation*, Grabowski and Hall, pp. 102-109.

10. Valerie DeBenedette, "OTC Status for Nicotine Gum Not in the Cards," *Medical Advertising News*, Vol. 4, No. 21, December 15, 1985.

11. Nicorette Package Insert, Merrill-Dow, 1984; M. A. H. Russell and M. J. Jarvis, "Theoretical Background and Clinical Use of Nicotine Chewing Gum," in *Pharmacological Adjuncts in Smoking Cessation*, Grabowski and Hall, p. 127.

12. Jarvis et al., "Randomized Controlled Trial of Nicotine Chewing Gum," *British Medical Journal*, Vol. 285, pp. 537-540, August 21, 1982.

13. Personal communication from M.A.H. Russell, June 12, 1986. Karl-Olov Fagerstrom and Bo Melin, "Nicotine Chewing Gum in Smoking Cessation," Grabowski and Hall, p. 102-109.

14. John R. Hughes et al., "Physical Dependence on Nicotine in Gum," *Journal of the American Medical Association*, Vol. 255, No. 23, June 20, 1986.

15. C. Everett Koop, *The Health Consequences of Smoking: Nicotine Addiction*, A report of the Surgeon General, U.S. Department of Health and Human Services, 1988, pp. 480–481; M.A.H. Russell, Martin J. Jarvis, et al., "Nicotine Replacement in Smoking Cessation," *Journal of the American Medical Association*, June 19, 1987, pp. 3262–3265.

16. Turner, James E., phone interview with the author, May 6, 1988. Accrding to Turner, all rights to the Favor product are now owned by the Swedish pharmacological firm A.B. Leo, the manufacturer of Nicorette. Leo and Advanced Tobacco Products are currently involved in a joint venture to develop and market an improved version of the Favor inhaler. For more information contact James E. Turner, CEO, Advanced Tobacco Products, Route 27, Box 330-P, San Antonio TX 78245, (512)677-8611.

17. Personal communication from M.A.H. Russell, June 12, 1986.

18. Jed E. Rose et al., "Transdermal Nicotine Reduces Cigarette Craving and Nicotine Preference," *Clinical Pharmacology and Therapeutics*, Vol. 38, No. 4, pp. 450-456, October 1985; J. E. Rose et al., "Transdermal Administration of Nicotine," *Drug and Alcohol Dependence*, Vol. 13, pp. 209-213, 1984.

19. Jed E. Rose, "The Role of Upper Airway Stimulation in Smoking," in *Nicotine Replacement: A Critical Evaluation*, Alan R. Liss, Inc., New York, NY, 1988, pp. 95–106; Jed Rose, phone interview with the author, May 6, 1988. For further information on aerosol sprays for smokers, contact Jed E. Rose, Ph.D., Veteran's Administration Medical Center at Brentwood, Building 206, Room 29, Los Angeles CA 90073, (213)824-4420.

20. C. Everett Koop, *The Health Consequences of Smoking: Nicotine Addiction*. A report of the Surgeon General, U.S. Department of Health and Human Services, 1988, pp. 479–480; Personal communication from M.A.H. Russell, June 12, 1986.

Chapter 10

1. Personal communication from Edward Lichtenstein, Professor of Psychology, University of Oregon, June 13, 1986.

2. Alexander H. Glassman, Wynn K. Jackson, B. Timothy Walsh, and Bob Rosenfeld, "Cigarette Craving, Smoking Withdrawal, and Clonidine," *Science*, Vol. 226, pp. 864-866, November 16, 1984; "Drug Eases Cigarette Craving," *Medical World News*, January 14, 1985, pp. 29, 33.

3. Joe and Teresa Graedon, *The People's Pharmacy* (revised edition), St. Martin's Press, 1985, New York, p. 313.

4. These guidelines are adapted, with permission, from Brian G. Danaher and Edward Lichtenstein, *Become an Ex-Smoker*,

Prentice-Hall, Englewood Cliffs, NJ, 1978. Many thanks to Edward Lichtenstein for reviewing this material.

5. Edward Lichtenstein and Russell Glasgow, "Rapid Smoking: Side Effects and Safeguards," *Journal of Consulting and Clinical Psychology*, Vol. 45, pp. 815-821, 1977; David P. L. Sachs, quoted in "Rapid Smoking Helps Patients Kick the Habit," *Internal Medicine News*, Vol. 14, No. 16, August 1981; Edward Lichtenstein, "The Smoking Problem: A Behavioral Perspective," *Journal of Consulting and Clinical Psychology*, Vol. 50, No. 6, pp. 804-819, 1982.

6. Signing up as a *Medical Self-Care* subscriber can be an important part of a commitment to take better care of yourself. We've arranged for a special offer for readers of *The No-Nag, No-Guilt, Do-It-Your-Own-Way Guide to Quitting Smoking:* A year's subscription to *Medical Self-Care* for only $11.97, several dollars off the regular subscription price. You need send no money now, just send your name and address to *Medical Self-Care*, P. O. Box 717, Inverness, CA 94937, or call (415) 663-8462 to sign up for a one-year subscription. You'll be billed later.

Chapter 11

1. Personal communication from Neil E. Grunberg, August 1986. Dr. Grunberg is Associate Professor of Medical Physiology, Uniformed Services University of the Health Sciences, Bethesda, Maryland.

2. R. C. Trahair, "Giving Up Cigarettes: 222 Case Studies," *Medical Journal of Australia*, Vol. 1, pp. 929-932, 1967; Thomas J. Coates and Virginia C. Li, "Does Smoking Cessation Lead to Weight Gain?" *American Journal of Public Health*, Vol. 73, No. 11, 1983, pp. 1303-1304; Jeffrey T. Wack and Judith Rodin, "Smoking and Its Effects on Body Weight and the Systems of Caloric Regulation," *American Journal of Clinical Nutrition*, Vol. 35, pp. 366-380, 1982; Peter H. Blitzer et al., "The Effect of Smoking Cessation on Body Weight," *Journal of Chronic Diseases*, Vol. 30, pp. 415-429, 1977.

3. Personal communication from Neil E. Grunberg, June 1986.

4. Arden G. Christen and Kenneth H. Cooper, "Strategic Withdrawal from Cigarette Smoking," *CA: A Cancer Journal for Clinicians*, Vol. 29, No. 2, March/April 1979.

5. Neil E. Grunberg, "The Effects of Nicotine and Cigarette

Smoking on Food Consumption and Taste Preferences,'' *Journal of Addictive Behaviors*, Vol. 7, No. 4, pp. 317-331, 1982; D. Perlick, *The Withdrawal Syndrome: Nicotine Addiction and the Effects of Stopping Smoking in Heavy and Light Smokers*, doctoral dissertation, Department of Psychology, Columbia University, New York, 1977; personal communication from Neil E. Grunberg, June 1986.

6. William A. Check, ''Medical News: Smoking, Eating, and Nicotine,'' *Journal of the American Medical Association*, Vol. 247, No. 17, May 7, 1982, p. 2338; R. L. Burse et al., *Effects of Cigarette Smoking on Body Weight, Energy Expenditure, Appetite, and Endocrine Function*, U.S. Army Medical Research and Development Command, Fort Detrick, Frederick, Maryland, March 1982; A. Keys, ''Smoking, Lung Function, and Body Weight,'' *British Medical Journal*, Vol. 286, No. 6380, pp. 1823-1824, June 4, 1983.

7. ''Study Links Smoking and Weight,'' *The New York Times*, January 21, 1986, p. 18.

8. Jeffrey T. Wack and Judith Rodin, ''Smoking and Its Effects on Body Weight and the Systems of Caloric Regulation,'' *The American Journal of Clinical Nutrition*, Vol. 35, pp. 366-380, February 1982.

9. Robert M. Carney and Andrew P. Goldberg, ''Weight Gain After Cessation of Cigarette Smoking,'' *The New England Journal of Medicine*, Vol. 310, pp. 614-616, March 8, 1984.

10. B. Nemery et al., ''Smoking, Lung Function, and Body Weight,'' *British Medical Journal,''* Vol. 286, pp. 249-251, January 22, 1983.

11. T. A. Burling et al., ''Techniques Used by Smokers During Contingency Motivated Smoking Reduction,'' *Addictive Behaviors*, Vol. 7, No. 4, pp. 397-401, 1982.

12. David R. Jacobs and Sara Gottenborg, ''Smoking and Weight: The Minnesota Lipid Research Clinic,'' *American Journal of Public Health*, Vol. 71, No. 4, April 1981, pp. 391-396.

13. Neil Grunberg, ''The Effects of Nicotine and Cigarette Smoking on Food Consumption and Taste Preferences,'' *Addictive Behaviors*, Vol. 7, No. 4, pp. 317-331, 1982; Neil Grunberg, as quoted in Sally Squires, ''Sweet Smell of Smoke,'' *Austin American-Statesman*, January 6, 1985.

14. ''Weight Control Guidance in Smoking Cessation'' (pamphlet), The American Heart Association, Dallas, Texas, no date.

15. Alice Kahn, ''The All New Feminist No-Weight-Loss-Diet,'' *Medical Self-Care*, No. 21, Summer 1983, pp. 13-16.

16. Kim Chernin, *The Obsession: Reflections on the Tyranny of Slenderness*, Harper & Row, New York, 1982.

17. William Bennett and Joel Guren, *The Dieter's Dilemma*, Basic Books, New York, 1982.

Other sources for this chapter include: Ronald S. Manley and Frederick J. Boland, ''Side-Effects and Weight Gain Following a Smoking Cessation Program,'' *Addictive Behaviors*, Vol. 8, pp. 375-380, 1983; D. R. Powell and B. S. McCann, ''The Effects of a Multiple Treatment Program and Maintenance Procedures on Smoking Cessation,'' *Preventive Medicine*, Vol. 10, pp. 94-104, 1981. Special thanks to Dr. Neil E. Grunberg for his many helpful comments on this chapter.

Chapter 12

1. Saul Shiffman et al., ''Preventing Relapse in Ex-Smokers: A Self-Management Approach,'' in G. Alan Marlatt and Judith R. Gordon, *Relapse Prevention: Maintenance Strategies in the Treatment of Addictive Behaviors*, The Guilford Press, New York, 1985, pp. 472-520.

2. Ibid.

3. Ibid.

4. Ibid.

5. L. L. DeLoach, *Adolescent Initiation Into Cigarette Use: A Test of Two Theories*, doctoral dissertation, University of South Florida, Tampa, University Microfilms International 84-27957, August 1984; David L. Geisinger, *Kicking It: The New Way to Stop Smoking Permanently*, Signet Books/New American Library, New York, 1978.

6. Daniel J. Levinson et al., *The Seasons of a Man's Life*, Ballantine Books, New York, 1978.

7. Figure 12-1 was developed by the author, and was modeled after a somewhat similar graphic approach used by P. Elias Duryea et al. in ''Cognitive Perceptions of Importance in Students' Decisions About Smoking,'' *Health Education*, Vol. 12, No. 5, pp. 4-8, September/October 1981.

8. Levinson et al., pp. 192-199.

9. Levinson et al., pp. 192-193.

10. R. B. Friedlander, *The Helper-Therapy Principle in a Smoking Cessation Program*, doctoral dissertation, University of

Texas, Lubbock, Texas, University Microfilms International 83-02160, August 1982.

11. John S. Tamerin, "The Psychodynamics of Quitting in a Group Setting," *American Journal of Psychiatry*, Vol. 129, pp. 589-595, 1972.

12. Stanton Peele with Archie Brodsky, *Love and Addiction*, Signet Books/New American Library, New York, 1975, pp. 59-61.

13. Levinson et al., pp. 218-221.

14. Arden G. Christen and Kenneth H. Cooper, "Strategic Withdrawal from Cigarette Smoking," *CA: A Cancer Journal for Clinicians*, Vol. 29, No. 2, March/April 1979, p. 104.

15. Elaine Richard and Ann C. Shepard, "Giving Up Smoking: A Lesson in Loss Theory," *American Journal of Nursing*, April 1981, pp. 755-757; Christen and Cooper, pp. 96-107.

16. E. K. Schmookler, *A Study of Spontaneous Smoking Cessation*, doctoral dissertation, University of California, Berkeley, University Microfilms International, 84-00642, 1982.

17. The table of potential relapse crisis situations is adapted, with permission, from a similar table in Saul Shiffman et al., "Preventing Relapse in Ex-Smokers: A Self-Management Approach," in Marlatt and Gordon, op. cit.

18. The table of active and internal responses is adapted, with permission, from a similar table in Saul Shiffman et al., "Preventing Relapse in Ex-Smokers: A Self-Management Approach," in Alan G. Marlatt and Judith R. Gordon, *Relapse Prevention*, Guilford Press, New York, 1985, pp. 472-520.

Appendix I

1. Arden G. Christen and Kenneth H. Cooper, "Strategic Withdrawal from Cigarette Smoking," *CA: A Cancer Journal for Clinicians*, March/April 1979, pp. 96-107.

2. Personal communication from Karen Pryor, April 1986.

3. *Don't Shoot the Dog: The New Art of Teaching and Training*, Bantam Books, 1984.

Other sources for this appendix include: S. Cohen, "Alternatives to Adolescent Drug Abuse," *Journal of the American Medical Association*, Vol. 238, pp. 1561-1562, 1977; D. Oken, "Tobacco Addiction and Compassion," *Journal of the American Medical Association*, Vol. 253, No. 20, p. 2958, May 24-31, 1984;

Marcia Gammeter and Steve Barker, "Help a Friend—Adopt a Smoker" (press release, no date), Lemar Laboratories, Atlanta, GA; Irving L. Janis, "The Role of Social Support in Adherence to Stressful Decisions," *American Psychologist*, February 1983, pp. 143-160; Roy J. Shephard et al., "Reinforcement of a Smoking Withdrawal Program," *Canadian Journal of Public Health*, Vol. 64, March/April 1973, pp. S42-S51.

Appendix II

See Milton E. Eisen and E. Cuyler Hammond, "The Effect of Smoking on Packed Cell Volume, Red Blood Cell Counts, Hemoglobin, and Platelet Count," *Canadian Medical Association Journal*, Vol. 75, pp. 520-523, September 15, 1956; Verner J. Knott and Peter H. Venables, "EEG Correlates of Non-Smokers, Smokers, Smoking, and Smoking Deprivation," *Psychophysiology*, Vol. 14, pp. 150-156, 1977; G. S. Tell et al., "The Relationship of White Cell Count, Platelet Count, and Hematocrit to Cigarette Smoking in Adolescents," *Circulation*, Vol. 72, No. 5, pp. 971-974, November 1985; *Drug Effects Can Go Up in Smoke*, HEW Publication No. (FDA) 79-3086, March 1979, Reprinted from the *FDA Consumer*, March 1979; David S. Sobel and Tom Ferguson, *The People's Book of Medical Tests*, Summit Books, New York, 1985.

Appendix III

See Arthur G. Lipman, "How Smoking Interferes with Drug Therapy," *Modern Medicine*, August 1985, pp. 141-142; Joan Houghton et al., "Pharmacist's Role in Smoking Cessation," American Pharmacy, Vol. NS 26, No. 7, pp. 494-506, July 1986; E. J. S. Boyd et al., "Smoking Impairs Therapeutic Gastric Inhibition," *Lancet*, January 15, 1983, pp. 95-97; *Drug Effects Can Go Up in Smoke*, HEW Publication No. (FDA) 79-3086, March 1979, reprinted from the *FDA Consumer*, March 1979; Jytte Jensen et al., "Cigarette Smoking, Serum Estrogens, and Bone Loss During Estrogen-Replacement Therapy Early After Menopause," *The New England Journal of Medicine*, Vol. 313, No. 16, pp. 973-975, October 17, 1985; Peter W. F. Wilson et al., "Postmenopausal Estrogen Use, Cigarette Smoking, and Cardiovascular Morbidity in Women Over 50," *The New England Journal of Medicine*, Vol. 313, No. 17, pp. 1038-1043, October 24, 1985.

Index

ABOUT THE AUTHOR

Award-winning medical writer **Tom Ferguson, M.D.** is president of the Center for Self-Care Studies in Austin, Texas.

Dr. Ferguson received his M.D. from the Yale University School of Medicine. He was the founding editor of **Medical Self-Care** magazine and is founder and editor-at-large of the **SelfCare Catalog.** He has served for many years as medical editor of the **Whole Earth Catalog.**

His books include **Medical Self-Care: Access to Health Tools, The People's Book of Medical Tests, The No-Nag, No-Guilt, Do-It-Your-Own-Way Guide to Quitting Smoking,** and **Helping Smokers Get Ready to Quit: A New Approach to the Toughest Problem in Health Promotion** (see p. 256).

Dr. Ferguson has received the National Educational Press Association's **Distinguished Achievement Award** for his writings on raising health-responsible children. He received the **Lifetime Extension Award** for his writings on the rapidly expanding area of self-help and self-care. His work has been cited by author John Naisbitt in his book **Megatrends** as representing "the essence of the shift from institutional help to self-help." He has appeared on **60 Minutes, The Today Show,** and the **Cable News Network** as an expert on self-help, self-care, and smoking and has done hundreds of other radio, TV, and newspaper interviews.

He is a popular speaker and workshop leader for professional and lay audiences from coast to coast. His most popular presentations include "Health in the Information Age," "Empowerment: The Heart of Wellness," "Raising Health-Responsible Children," and "Empowering the Smoker: A Positive Approach to Smoking Cessation." He provides consulting and training services to health care institutions and corporations planning stop-smoking programs and implementing workplace smoking policies.

Dr. Ferguson lives in Austin, Texas, with his wife, his daughter, and their two cats.

For more information on Dr. Ferguson's books and presentations, please write or call the Center for Self-Care Studies, 3805 Stevenson Avenue, Austin, TX 78703. (512) 472-1333.